Contemporary Diagnosis and Management of *Thyroid Disorders*®

John F. Wilber, MD
Professor of Medicine
Division of Endocrinology, Diabetes, and Nutrition
University of Maryland School of Medicine
Baltimore, Maryland

First Edition

Published by Handbooks in Health Care Co.
Newtown, Pennsylvania, USA

Dedication

To my wife, Joan, with greatest appreciation for her enduring support.

This book has been prepared and is presented as a service to the medical community. The information provided reflects the knowledge, experience, and personal opinions of John F. Wilber, MD, Professor of Medicine, Division of Endocrinology, Diabetes, and Nutrition, University of Maryland School of Medicine, Baltimore, Maryland.

This book is not intended to replace or to be used as a substitute for the complete prescribing information prepared by each manufacturer for each drug. Because of possible variations in drug indications, in dosage information, in newly described toxicities, in drug/drug interactions, and in other items of importance, reference to such complete prescribing information is definitely recommended before any of the drugs discussed are used or prescribed.

International Standard Book Number: 1-884065-31-7

Library of Congress Catalog Card Number: 98-70975

 For information, write Handbooks in Health Care, 3 Terry Drive, Suite 201, Newtown, Pennsylvania 18940, (215) 860-9600.
Web site: www.HHCbooks.com

Contents

Chapter 1

The Normal Thyroid Gland: Structure and Function

The thyroid gland is the largest endocrine structure in humans. It secretes two hormones, T_4 (L-3,5,3',5'-tetraiodothyronine) and T_3 (L-3,5,3'-triiodothyronine). T_3 and T_4 regulate oxidative metabolism and heat production, and contribute importantly to somatic growth.[1]

The thyroid is located in front of the trachea, midway between the sternal notch and the thyroid cartilage (Figure 1-1). It originates as an evagination from the base of the tongue, and grows downward and anteriorly to form two fusiform-shaped lobes on each side of the trachea, connected by the isthmus. The pyramidal lobe is a small vertical extension from the isthmus in the midline.[2] Microscopic examination of a normal thyroid gland reveals numerous follicles containing a centrally located pink-staining material, the colloid, where iodinated thyroglobulin is stored.

The synthesis of T_4 and T_3 by thyroid follicular cells involves several steps. First, iodide ions are transported actively across the basement membrane against a 50:1 electrochemical gradient. Next, iodide ions are oxidized and incorporated into monoiodotyrosine (MIT) and diiodotyrosine (DIT) residues within the thyroglobulin tetrameric protein. Two DITs can couple to form T_4, and one MIT and one DIT can couple to form T_3 moieties in thyroglobulin (Tg). Tg is hydrolyzed by thyroid-stimulating hormone (TSH) stimulation to release T_4, T_3, MIT, and DIT. Iodide ions from unused MIT and DIT are conserved through an intrathyroidal *deiodinase* system.[3]

Inborn errors of certain steps in thyroid hormonogenesis (eg, iodide transport, iodide organification) may result in congenital, goitrous hypothyroidism.

Thyroid Hormones in Circulation: The Protein Binding System

Thyroid hormones are insoluble at pH 7.4 and are rendered soluble in serum by binding to three proteins: thyroid-binding globulin (TBG, an inter-α-globulin), thyroxin-binding prealbumin (TBPA, transthyretin), and albumin itself.[4] Between 70% and 75% of T_4 is bound to TBG, 15% to 20% to TBPA, and the remainder is associated with albumin. T_3, in contrast, is carried primarily on TBG (70% to 75%), with the remainder on albumin. Although molar T_4 concentrations in serum are 75 to 100 times higher than those of T_3, T_3 is the biologically important hormone at the nuclear level (intracellularly), where it modulates gene transcription. Eighty-five percent of circulating T_3 comes from the peripheral monodiiodination of T_4 to T_3 in the liver and in other structures by a 5' *deiodinase* enzyme, rather than by direct secretion of T_3 from the thyroid itself.

Control of Thyroid Function

The constancy of circulating T_4 and T_3 is achieved by a dynamic, negative feedback system involving hypothalamic thyrotropin-releasing hormone (TRH), pituitary TSH, and T_4 and T_3 from the thyroid gland (Figure 1-2).[5] TSH secretion is activated by TRH. After TSH stimulation, thyroid hormones inhibit both the actions of TRH on the pituitary and the formation and secretion of TRH from the hypo-

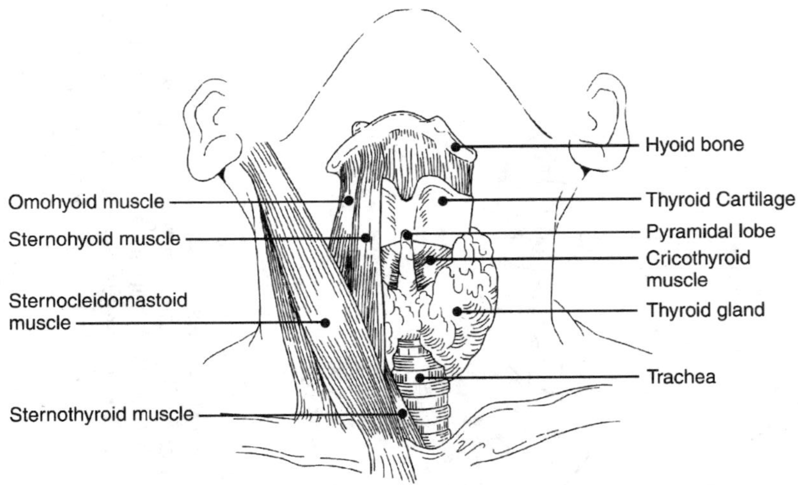

Figure 1-1: Gross anatomy of the human thyroid gland, anterior view. (Used with permission from: *Basic and Clinical Endocrinology*. Greenspan FS, Strewler GS, eds. Stanford, CT, Appleton & Lange, 1997).

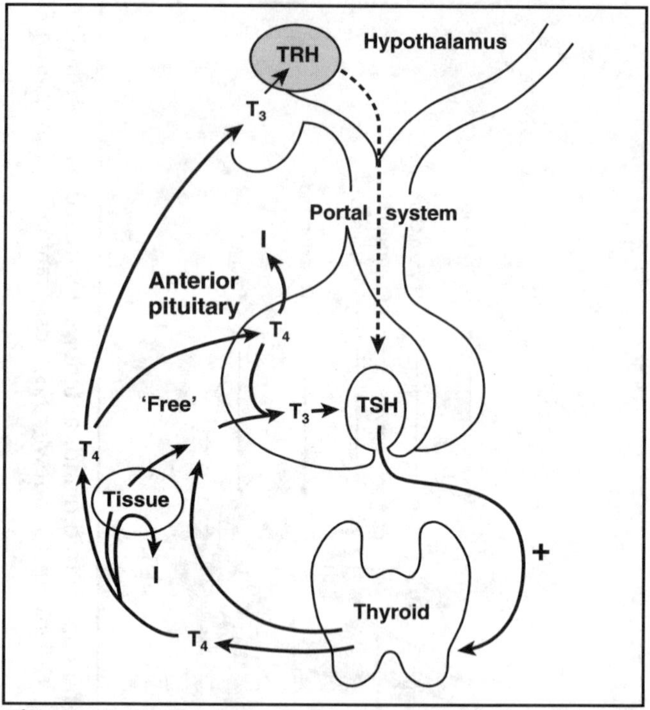

Figure 1-2: The hypothalamic-pituitary-thyroid axis. Hypothalamic TRH stimulates the synthesis and secretion of pituitary TSH, which in turn stimulates thyroidal growth and thyroid hormone secretion of T_4 and T_3. T_3 feeds back negatively at both the pituitary level and at the hypothalamic level by decreasing TRH production and secretion. (Used with permission from: *Basic and Clinical Endocrinology*. Greenspan FS, Strewler GS, eds. Stanford, CT, Appleton & Lange, 1997).

thalamus. TSH is the main regulator of thyroid gland growth, hormonogenesis, and hormone secretion. In addition, the thyroid gland has the unique ability to regulate itself.[6] Thus, in iodine deficiency, the thyroid gland can increase its iodide uptake and the intrathyroidal ratio of T_3 to T_4. Conversely, excess iodide can inhibit thyroid organification itself, a process commonly termed the Wolff-Chaikoff effect.[1] In addition to inhibiting thyroid hormone synthesis, pharmacologic doses of iodide can also inhibit hormone release. This property is exploited in the therapy of hyperthyroidism (see Chapters 3 and 4).

Pituitary TSH initiates its actions by binding to a specific, 7-transmembrane spanning receptor in the thyroid cell plasma membrane, which interacts with the *adenylate cyclase* signal transduction system.[7] TSH receptor mutations can lead to constitutive activation of thyroid nodules, which causes hyperthyroidism, as well as to inactivation of the receptor, which leads to hypothyroidism.[2]

Two other thyroid-stimulating proteins can play a role in thyroid function in both health and disease. During normal pregnancy, the concentration of human chorionic gonadotropin (hCG) rises to a maximum at 12 weeks, and plasma TSH reciprocally reaches a nadir. This suggests that hCG shares cross-biologic activity with TSH on the thyroid gland, although the activity ratio is 1:10,000 (hCG/TSH). Patients with trophoblastic malignancies, including hydatidiform moles and choriocarcinomas, can develop thyrotoxicosis from hCG stimulation of the thyroid if hCG levels are extremely high. In Graves' disease, there is an antibody (IgG) directed against TSH receptor epitopes. This thyroid-stimulating immunoglobulin (TSI) stimulates the thyroid gland and is responsible for hyperthyroidism in Graves' disease.[5]

Other factors important in thyroid regulation include glucocorticoids, which can inhibit thyroid function at both the pituitary and hypothalamic levels, and dopamine, which can inhibit both TSH and TRH secretion. Thus, these effects provide a pathophysiology for the central hypothyroidism syndromes that occur in the intensive care unit, where both corticosteroids and L-dopa are frequently used.

Finally, certain pharmacologic agents in food can inhibit thyroid hormone synthesis, and can lead to hypothyroidism.[8] The thionamide goitrogens, propylthiouracil and methimazole, used in pharmacotherapy for hyperthyroidism, can produce hypothyroidism. Other molecules also have antithyroid activity, including lithium, which, like iodide, can inhibit thyroid hormone release. This effect of lithium accounts for the hypothyroidism in patients with bipolar disorders undergoing lithium treatment. Several other antithyroid chemicals occur naturally in food, such as the Cruciferae plant family, which includes cabbage, turnips, rutabaga, and kale. Thiocyanate is one molecule responsible for the goitrogenic effects of these foods, especially in cabbage leaves. The pathogenetic role of these dietary goitrogens is not completely established, but their effects largely depend on the concomitant intake of environmental iodide. If iodine is insufficient, goitrous hypothyroidism can develop. Thus, this is almost nonexistent in the United States. Finally, certain sulfur-containing goitrogens of mineral origin are important contributors to the development of endemic goiter in other countries, such as Colombia, South America.[3]

Thyroid Hormone Action

Free T_3 and free T_4 are transported by passive diffusion or by specific carriers, through cell membranes, to bind to specific thyroid hormone receptors in the cell nucleus. Within many cells, T_4 is converted to T_3 by 5' deiodinase, indicating that T_4 is a prohormone for T_3, the active intracellular hormone. Nuclear T_3 receptor proteins have four splicing variants, $\alpha1$, $\alpha2$, $\beta1$, and $\beta2$.[9] These T_3 receptors, like those for steroid hormones, have a ligand-independent domain at the amino terminus, a central DNA-binding domain with a 'zinc' finger, and a specific ligand-binding domain for T_3 at the C terminus. Because TR-$\alpha2$ has an altered-ligand binding domain that is unable to bind

T_3, TR-α2 not only does not mediate T_3 actions, but may inhibit T_3 actions by 'dominant negative' mechanisms.[10] Thyroid hormone receptors act by forming as heterodimers with a related receptor protein, retinoid-x-receptor (RXR), whose ligand is 9-cis retinoic acid. TR-RXR heterodimers then bind to specific hormone recognition elements (TREs), located predominantly in the 5' flanking region of T_3-responsive genes. Because thyroid hormones require binding to receptors for their action, point mutations in the ligand-binding domain of TR receptors that prevent T_3 binding can cause the syndrome of 'thyroid hormone resistance' with high serum T_4 and T_3 concentrations. In selected instances, gene transcription is inhibited by T_3, as in pituitary TSH and hypothalamic TRH. These thyroid hormone receptors are close members of the larger 'superfamily' of nuclear receptors, including those for glucocorticoids, mineralocorticoids, estrogens, progesterone, testosterone, vitamin D, vitamin A, and retinoic acid-related ligands.

References

1. Braverman LE, Utiger RD, eds: Werner and Ingbar's *The Thyroid: A Fundamental and Clinical Text*, 7th ed. Philadelphia, Lippincott, 1996, pp 19-38.

2. Lindner HH: The thyroid gland. In: *Clinical Anatomy*. Appleton & Lange, 1989.

3. Eckholm R: Biosynthesis of thyroid hormones. *Int Rev Cytol* 1990;120:243.

4. Henneman G, Doctor R: Plasma transport proteins and their role in tissue delivery of thyroid hormone. In: Greer MA, ed. *The Thyroid Gland*. Martini L, ed. Comprehensive Endocrinology Series. New York, Raven Press, 1990, pp 79-101.

5. Utiger RD: The thyroid: physiology, thyrotoxicosis, hypothyroidism and the painful thyroid. In: Felig P, Baxter JD, Frohman LA, eds. *Endocrinology and Metabolism*, 3rd ed. New York, McGraw-Hill, 1995, pp 281-350.

6. Pisarev MA: Thyroid autoregulation. *J Endocrinol Invest* 1985;8:475-484.

7. Nagayama Y, Rapoport B: The thyrotropin receptor 25 years after its discovery: new insights after its molecular cloning. *Mol Endocrinol* 1992;6:145-156.

8. Wartofsky L, ed: The thyroid gland. In: Becker KL, ed. *Principles and Practice of Endocrinology and Metabolism*, 2nd ed. Philadelphia, Lippincott, 1995, pp 285-299.

9. Schwartz HL, Strait KA, Oppenheimer JH: Molecular mechanisms of thyroid hormone action. A physiologic perspective. *Clin Lab Med* 1993;13:543-561.

10. Lazar MA, Chin WW: Nuclear thyroid hormone receptors. *J Clin Invest* 1990;86:1777-1782.

Chapter 2

Physical Examination of the Thyroid Gland

For optimal examination of the thyroid gland,[1] the patient should be seated in a well-lit environment. A glass of water should be available to facilitate swallowing. The thyroid gland is first observed anteriorly. Upon swallowing, the gland should move upward, and, at this time, enlargement or nodular abnormalities may be seen. The patient is then asked to swallow while the examiner palpates the gland from behind, placing the middle three fingers on each lobe just below the cricoid cartilage (Figure 2-1). Goiter size can be measured with a 'goitergram.' Thyroid gland margins are first marked with a ballpoint pen. This ink image is then transferred to a piece of filter paper moistened with alcohol. After making the image transfer, the ink marks are removed from the neck with an alcohol swab. Goiter size can also be quantified by ultrasonography, or by neck circumference measurements taken with a standard tape measure.

Additional maneuvers can help clarify the significance of identified thyroid abnormalities. The inferior pole of each thyroid lobe should be identified by palpation during swallowing, which insures the absence of a substernal goiter. When a nodule is identified in or near the midline, upward movement of this mass after tongue protrusion is characteristic of thyroglossal duct cysts. Careful palpa-

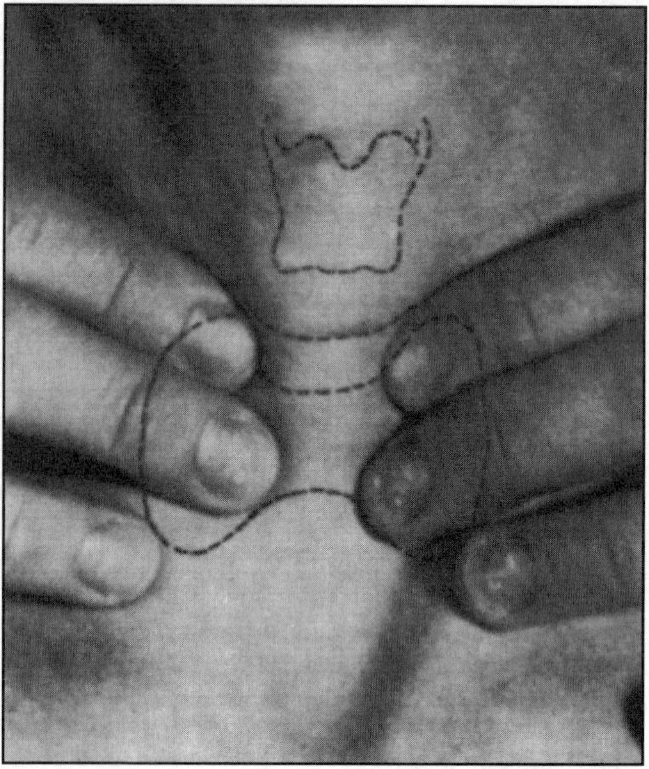

Figure 2-1: Correct physical examination of the human thyroid gland. The cricoid cartilage is located, and the index fingers are placed so that the superior portion rests against the inferior portion of the cricoid cartilage. The inferior portion of the index fingers is over the superior portion of the thyroid gland. The second and third fingers are then placed over the remainder of the thyroid gland to evaluate its size, contour, consistency, and possible adherence to surrounding structures. If the patient has difficulty swallowing during the examination, he or she is instructed to swallow a small amount of water provided by the physician to facilitate deglutition.

tion should be done to characterize the features and texture of the thyroid. The thyroid gland is typically *softer* than normal in Graves' thyrotoxicosis because of enhanced blood flow, and *firmer* than normal in chronic lymphocytic thyroiditis (Hashimoto's disease). An enlarged pyramidal lobe indicates generalized thyroid involvement, such as in Graves' disease or chronic lymphocytic thyroiditis.

Associated cervical lymphadenopathy should always be examined when nodules are present. If a malignant thyroid nodule is identified by fine-needle aspiration biopsy, palpation should include not only the thyroid itself, but also the skull, for potential lytic metastatic foci. Other features that suggest a possible malignant nodular lesion include rapid growth, calcification, or the development of hoarseness. 'Thyroid' nodules also may represent lesions from other origins, such as medullary carcinoma from thyroid C cells, metastatic nonthyroid cancer (eg, lymphoma), and, rarely, parathyroid carcinomas and granulomatous infections (see Chapter 8).

Reference

1. Larson PR, Davies TF, Hay ID: The thyroid gland. In: Wilson FD, Foster DW, Kronenberg HM, et al, eds. *Williams' Textbook of Endocrinology*, 9th ed. Philadelphia, WB Saunders Co, 1998, pp 389-516.

Chapter 3

Graves' Disease: The Most Common Cause of Thyrotoxicosis

Graves' disease is the most common and most important form of thyrotoxicosis (Figure 3-1). It occurs most often in the 3rd and 4th decades, and it is approximately 9 times more frequent in females than in males. The symptoms of Graves' disease include diffuse thyromegaly, thyrotoxicosis, ophthalmopathy (exophthalmos), and pretibial myxedema (dermopathy). Graves' disease has an autoimmune pathophysiology that is not completely understood. About 50% of relatives have circulating thyroid autoantibodies to thyroglobulin and thyroid *peroxidase*, indicating a strong familial predisposition.[1]

Pathophysiology

Thyroid-stimulating antibodies are generated by T-lymphocytes that become sensitized to certain thyroid epitopes. Stimulated β-lymphocytes secrete antibodies, including thyroid-stimulating immunoglobulin (TSI), which is directed to the thyroid-stimulating hormone (TSH) receptor on the thyroid cell surface. This antibody can be identified in more than 90% of patients with Graves' disease.[2-4] IgG antibodies that inhibit TSH binding to the TSH receptor may also occur in Graves' disease (TSH

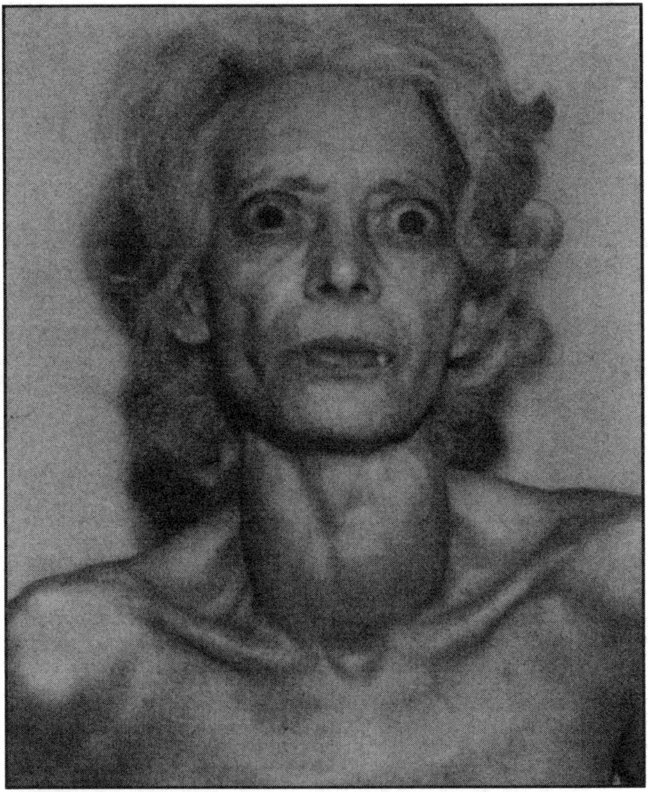

Figure 3-1: Thyrotoxicosis due to Graves' disease. Note the stare with lid retraction, the atrophy of shoulder girdle musculature, and the diffuse enlargement of the thyroid gland in the anterior neck.

receptor-binding-inhibiting immunoglobulins [TBII]). When these predominate over TSI activity, primary hypothyroidism occurs instead of thyrotoxicosis. Thyrotoxicosis usually is the sole manifestation of Graves' disease. However, patients sometimes present initially with hypothyroidism, later becoming thyrotoxic. Moreover, new-

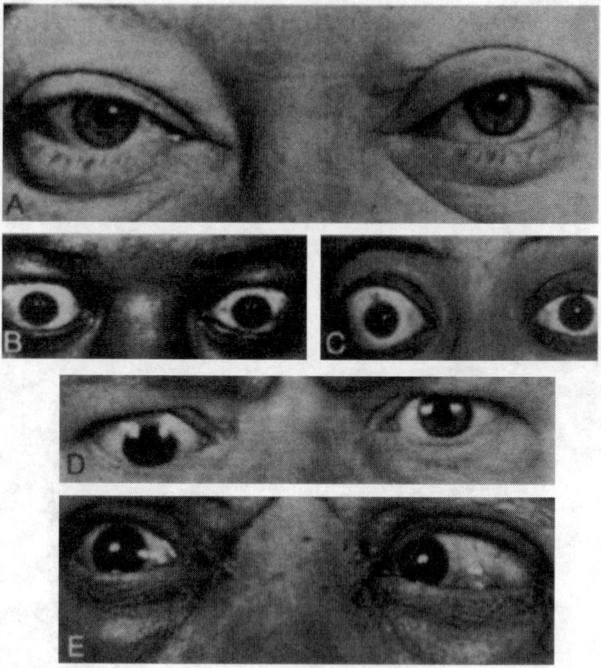

borns may be hypothyroid for a few weeks postpartum, manifesting thyrotoxicosis later as the thyroid-blocking, maternally derived antibodies are cleared.[5]

Graves' disease, like lymphocytic thyroiditis, may emerge postpartum after the immunosuppressive effects of normal pregnancy dissipate. Similarly, Graves' disease can be activated after corticosteroid withdrawal.

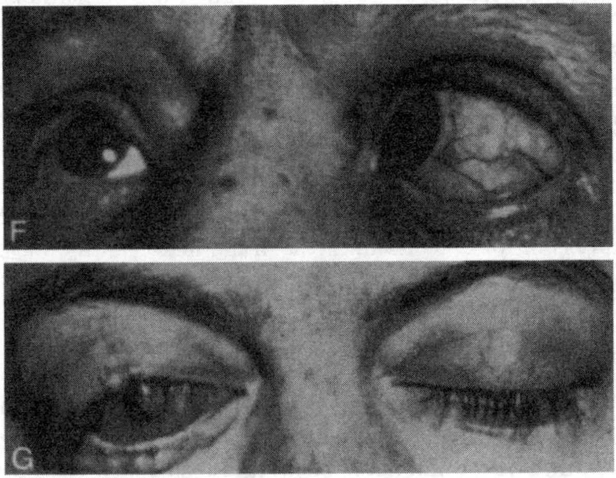

Figure 3-2: Graves' orbitopathy. A, palpebral edema. B, the widening of palpebral fissures. C, unequal degrees of exophthalmos. D, unilateral lid retraction. E, palpebral swelling, with paralysis of the right external rectus muscle. F, conjunctival infection and chemosis with ophthalmoplegia. G, failure to approximate lids because of marked exophthalmos, leading to corneal scarring and panophthalmitis. (Used with permission from: *Williams' Texbook of Endocrimology.* Wilson JD, Foster DW, Kronenberg HM, et al, eds. Philadelphia, WB Saunders Co, 1998).

No evidence suggests that psychologic stress can trigger Graves' disease.

Other extrathyroid manifestations of Graves' disease may include features of generalized immune activation, including generalized lymphadenopathy, splenomegaly, thymus enlargement, and autoimmune vitiligo.[6] Exophthalmos may occur in euthyroid individuals ('euthyroid'

Graves' disease), further emphasizing the independence of orbitopathy upon excess circulating thyroid hormones (Figure 3-2). Moreover, exophthalmos is not seen in other forms of hyperthyroidism, such as thyrotoxicosis factitia from ingestion of excessive L-thyroxine.

Many features of thyrotoxic Graves' disease, including systolic hypertension, sinus tachycardia, tremor, diaphoresis, lid lag, and stare, are likely caused by enhanced expression of catecholamines. In the heart, an increased number of adrenergic receptors have been shown to be increased in experimental thyrotoxicosis models.[1,7]

Clinical Signs and Symptoms

In young patients, the most common symptoms are nervousness, palpitations, hyperkinesis, hyperdefecation, sweating, heat tolerance, and weight loss despite a vigorous appetite. Diffuse thyromegaly is present, with a texture softer than normal because of increased blood flow. Proximal muscle weakness almost always is present; when testing quadricep strength by squatting, patients must be supported by the physician to prevent injury.

Cardiovascular and myopathic manifestations predominate in older individuals, while other symptoms frequent in younger patients can be masked.[8] Thus, the elderly may present only with palpitations, shortness of breath, tremor, and nervousness, and many other signs may be absent.

Graves' orbitopathy can be semiquantitatively classified by the mnemonic NOSPECS system, with classes 0 to 6. N represents *no* signs or symptoms; O is only signs, such as stare and lid lag; S designates symptoms of soft-tissue involvement; P signifies proptosis quantified by exophthalmometer; E is extraocular muscle involvement; C represents corneal involvement; and S represents sight loss with optic nerve involvement.[6]

Physical examination of the eye should begin with inspection for conjunctival edema (chemosis), signs of soft-tissue inflammation, and signs of extraocular myositis, detected by having the patient abduct the eye to permit examination of the contralateral, lateral rectus insertion. Extraocular myositis reveals a beefy, red, enlarged muscle, classic and unique in Graves' orbitopathy. Because Graves' disease is the most common cause of unilateral exophthalmos as well, it is important to distinguish this from other causes of proptosis. B-mode ultrasound or orbital computed tomography (CT) allow for recognition of enlarged muscles, which is the anatomic reason for globe displacement anteriorly.[9]

Thyroid dermopathy is manifested by thickening of the skin over the anterior shin, with purple papules over pruritic raised plaque. This occurs rarely (2% of Graves' patients). Pretibial myxedema invariably occurs in Graves' patients with exophthalmos and a very high TSI titer. The cause is unknown.

Laboratory findings in thyrotoxicosis include elevated free thyroxine, disproportionately elevated free T_3 over T_4, and markedly reduced serum TSH, usually below 0.05 µU/mL. The only other cause for such suppressed TSH would be secondary (pituitary) or tertiary (hypothalamic) hypothyroidism caused by low TSH. Such central hypothyroidism is easily distinguished from Graves' disease because signs of thyrotoxicosis and extrathyroid signs of Graves' disease are absent.[1,7]

The differential diagnosis in Graves' disease includes states with severe muscle atrophy, such as polymyositis. Hypokalemic periodic paralysis may be present, typically in Asian individuals. This syndrome resolves when thyrotoxicosis is treated. Patients with primary cardiac involvement (eg, refractory atrial fibrillation, high output failure) usually have no evidence of underlying heart disease. Cardiac manifestations are cured by treatment.[8] Diagnosis can be very difficult when older patients present with weight loss, small goiters, slow atrial fibrillation, and depression, the syndrome of 'apathetic hyperthyroidism.'

Rarely, women may present with amenorrhea. Thus, the diagnosis of hyperthyroidism requires a high degree of suspicion and appropriate laboratory studies. The syndrome of *familial dysalbuminemic hyperthyroxinemia* is caused by secretion of abnormal albumin-like proteins from the thyroid gland that preferentially bind T_4, but not T_3. This leads to a marked elevation in serum thyroxine, but free T_3 and T_4 concentrations are normal and TSH is not suppressed. Although T_4 concentrations may range from 50 to 100 μg/dL, and the normal TSH and serum T_3 rule out thyrotoxicosis.

Treatment of Graves' Disease

Ideally, therapy should be directed at the underlying etiology, but the present methods of treating autoimmunity are more dangerous than the thyrotoxicosis itself. The three main therapeutic options are antithyroid drug therapy, iodine 131 (^{131}I) therapy, and surgical removal of the thyroid.[10]

Antithyroid drug therapy is most useful in patients with small thyroid glands and mild, brief clinical manifestations. The two drugs used in the United States are methimazole (Tapazole®) and propylthiouracil (PTU). These are administered in initial doses of 30 to 60 mg/d and 300 to 600 mg/d, respectively. The spontaneous remission rate is approximately 30% in the first 3 to 12 months after beginning therapy. PTU, which is 10-fold less potent than methimazole on a molar basis, has the unique advantage of not only blocking thyroid hormone synthesis, but also blocking T_4-to-T_3 conversion when given in sufficiently high doses (>600 mg/d). Medical therapy for Graves' disease is difficult because a long period of observation is required before medical therapy is stopped, and the relapse rate is high.

A typical therapy is oral PTU, 100 to 200 mg every 8 hours. PTU only comes in 50-mg tablets, so 600 mg/d would require 12 extremely bitter pills. In contrast, methimazole in comparable doses (10 to 20 mg q 8 h) often can be given once a day in the morning. Methimazole tablets come in both 5 mg and 10 mg, and are not bitter. Methimazole is typically started with a 40-mg dose each morning for 2 months, and then gradually reduced to 5 to 10 mg/d for maintenance therapy while awaiting a potential spontaneous remission. If administration of antithyroid drugs induces hypothyroidism, the patient may be given 100 μg/d of thyroxine in conjunction with antithyroid therapy. Therapy usually is continued for 6 to 12 months or until sustained remission can be predicted, based on a reduction in thyroid gland size, and/or anti-TSH receptor antibody titers becoming much lower or detectable.

Side effects of antithyroid drugs are not common, but are potentially serious. Allergic reactions, including rash, occur in about 5% of patients, and bone marrow suppression occurs in less than 1%.[10] Agranulocytosis requires immediate cessation of therapy and institution of appropriate antibiotics. Fever and pharyngitis may accompany leukopenia; therefore, all patients should be instructed that if these symptoms occur, drug therapy should be stopped immediately and the managing physician should be consulted. Rarely (1/1,400), hepatocellular toxicity with jaundice may occur. This syndrome must be recognized early, when the process is completely reversible. Failure to stop therapy immediately may lead to total liver failure and the need for liver transplantation.

Surgical Therapy

Near-total thyroidectomy is appropriate for patients under 15 years of age, in patients with very large thyroid glands or multinodular goiters underlying Graves' disease, and in the second trimester of pregnancy if drug therapy fails. *Total* thyroidectomy is inappropriate because the parathyroid glands may be inadvertently extirpated. Ideally, approximately 1 g of thyroid tissue should be left on each side to prevent hypothyroidism and hypoparathyroidism. An additional, uncommon complication of surgery in about 1% of patients is interruption of the recurrent laryngeal nerve, which can result in hoarseness.

^{131}I Therapy

^{131}I therapy is the preferred treatment for most Graves' patients over 21. In patients without underlying heart disease, radioiodine can be given in doses of 80 to 120 μCi/g of estimated thyroid weight, adjusted to the uptake.[11] For example, if the thyroid uptake is 50%, the calculated dose of radioiodine must be doubled to deliver the appropriate dose (100%) to the thyroid. Because ^{131}I administration can induce irradiation injury (thyroiditis), with release of T_4 and T_3, patients with underlying heart disease or very severe thyrotoxicosis should be rendered euthyroid with antithyroid drugs before ^{131}I therapy. Antithyroid drugs must be stopped 1 week before administration of ^{131}I to ensure the expected ^{131}I organification. Moreover, a pregnancy test should be performed in all women of childbearing age, because pregnancy is a contraindication to ^{131}I administration. The only major complication of radioiodine therapy is hypothyroidism, occurring in 20% of subjects in the first year, and in 4% per year thereafter. Thus, patients must be followed carefully, because most will develop hypothyroidism by year 20 after ^{131}I. Increased cardiovascular and stroke mortality has been recently reported in patients with hyperthyroidism treated with ^{131}I. The role of ^{131}I in this complication is not clear, however, because mortality does *not* correlate with ^{131}I dosage.[10]

Ancillary Therapeutic Measures for Graves' Disease

In conjunction with antithyroid drugs (PTU, methimazole), β-adrenergic blocking agents are useful in controlling palpitations, tachycardia, tremulousness, nervousness, sweating, and anxiety.[1,7] Propranolol (Inderal®) can be given in daily divided doses of 40 to 160 mg. These symptoms also may be controlled with longer-acting β-blockers, such as metoprolol (Toprol-XL®).

Nonradioactive iodide is useful in blocking thyroid hormonogenesis, administered as sodium ipodate or iopanoic acid. Iodide ions inhibit both thyroid hormone production and thyroid hormone secretion, as well as peripheral conversion of T_4 to T_3. A dosage of 1 g daily can rapidly induce euthyroidism. Iodides should not be given before ^{131}I therapy, however, because ^{127}I precludes entry of radioiodine into the thyroid gland for several weeks. Patients with very large goiters and allergic reactions to antithyroid drugs can be treated with sodium ipodate in combination with β-blockers.

Therapeutic Choices

In the United States and Western Europe, ^{131}I therapy is the preferred treatment for Graves' disease. In Asia, antithyroid drug therapy is preferred. These two therapies are not mutually exclusive, however. Antithyroid drug therapy can be given to achieve euthyroidism before radioiodine or surgery is considered. After ^{131}I treatment for Graves' disease, methimazole or PTU can be reinstated to sustain euthyroidism until the effects of radiation are fully realized (4 to 6 months).[1,3,7]

Thyroid Storm

Thyroid storm can occur in all forms of thyrotoxicosis. It is characterized by tachycardia out of proportion to body temperature, and exaggerated manifestations of thyrotoxicosis in three systems: the central nervous system, the cardiovascular system, and the gastrointestinal system.[12] Thus, patients may develop severe congestive heart failure, often precipitated by tachyarrhythmias. The sensorium may be altered, including the development of coma. Finally, hepatocellular failure can develop with hepatomegaly and jaundice. Thyroid storm is precipitated by a number of conditions, including febrile illnesses, and surgery, including thyroid surgery itself. The molecular pathophysiology of this syndrome is not fully understood, but serum concentrations of T_4 and T_3 are *not* increased. Thus, researchers believe excessive expression of thyroid hormone reflects altered T_3-receptor interactions with thyroid recognition elements in T_3-responsive genes, which manifest enhanced transcription in response to T_3.

Thyroid storm requires aggressive recognition and management. Emergency therapy requires the administration of antithyroid drugs in high doses (methimazole, 30 mg q 6 h) to inhibit thyroid hormonogenesis. Methimazole must be administered at least 12 hours before iodide administration (eg, 1 g of intravenous sodium iodide over 24 hours) to prevent increased thyroid iodide concentrations, which enhance T_3 production and exacerbate hyperthyroidism.[12] In addition, glucocorticoids are administered to reduce T_4-to-T_3 conversion, and to treat the autoimmune process itself in Graves' disease, using hydrocortisone (50 mg q 6 h) or prednisone (10 mg q 6 h). Beta-blockers are given as well to control signs and symptoms (eg, tremor, tachycardia, hypertension) induced by increased adrenergic tone. In semicomatose or comatose patients, propranolol can be given, 1 mg/minute IV, or via a nasogastric, tube (60-80 mg q 4 h) to achieve β-adrenergic blockade. Additional measures include a cooling blanket and acetaminophen to lower temperature. Intravenous fluids, electrolytes, and B vitamins should be administered. Finally, underlying conditions that may have precipitated thyroid storm (eg, infections) should be treated (eg, with appropriate antibiotics). If standard medical therapies are not successful, plasmapheresis or hemodialysis can be employed.[12]

Thyrotoxicosis in Pregnancy

Hyperthyroidism in pregnancy is usually caused by Graves' disease. It can be associated with a number of complications, including fetal wastage, low birth weight, premature labor, hyperemesis gravidarum, maternal toxemia, and congestive heart failure.[13] In contrast, transient thyrotoxicosis, followed by transient hypothyroidism, occurs in about 5% of women postpartum (see Chapter 4).

Normal pregnancies and hyperthyroidism share some features that make diagnosis of thyrotoxicosis challenging. During normal pregnancy, the thyroid gland enlarges, particularly in iodine deficiency. There is evidence of hyperdynamic circulation and hypermetabolism, which usually peak around the 7th month.[13] Importantly, in both conditions, serum thyroxine and T_3 concentrations are increased, partly because thyroid-binding globulin (TBG) is elevated to raise TBG-binding capacity about 2-fold. Because radioiodine is contraindicated in pregnancy, the diagnosis of thyrotoxicosis in pregnancy requires measurement of the proportion of free thyroxine and free triiodothyronine in serum, and of TSH levels. It is important to understand that TSH can be partially suppressed, to 0.1 to 0.5 μU/mL during the 8th to the 14th week, because human chorionic gonadotropin (hCG) stimulation of the thyroid is associated with a reciprocal decline in TSH. Thus, when thyrotoxicosis is suspected, it is important to measure TSH with a *third*-generation ultrasensitive TSH assay. TSH levels at or below 0.1 μU/mL, accompanied by an elevation in free T_4 or free T_3, strongly suggest hyperthyroidism. The T_3:T_4 ratio usually is elevated in Graves' disease, in contrast to forms of hyperthyroidism such as thyroiditis, in which the thyroid is not stimulated by TSH or TSI and the T_3:T_4 ratio remains normal.

Management of hyperthyroidism during pregnancy is challenging. It must be managed because the frequency of spontaneous abortion is increased. The general principle is to use antithyroid drugs (PTU only, because methimazole is associated with a fetal scalp condition, aplasia cutis).[13] The goal is to administer as little PTU as possible to minimize excessive fetal thyroid PTU concentrations that can result in goiter in utero and fetal hypothyroidism. Thus, the mother's PTU dose can be titrated to achieve minimal thyrotoxicosis. This is usually achieved with doses of PTU between 50 and 100 mg/d. In patients in whom higher doses of PTU are required to maintain euthyroidism in pregnancy, subtotal thyroidectomy in the second trimester may be considered. As indicated below, although babies can develop goiters with intrauterine hypothyroidism from maternal treatment, they also are at risk for neonatal Graves' disease. The use of propranolol or other β-blockers in pregnancy is controversial because of reports of intrauterine growth retardation and neonatal hypoglycemia. In mothers with Graves' disease in remission when pregnancy is identified, or who already are taking antithyroid agents and want to become pregnant, antithyroid drugs (PTU) should be continued during pregnancy, or reinstituted if hyperthyroidism recurs. In such instances, ^{131}I therapy or surgery should be considered before pregnancy.

The therapy of Graves' disease in pregnancy, like that of Graves' disease in general, requires education of the patient, so that the risks and benefits of the alternatives are understood. Methimazole, but not PTU, can appear in breast milk; therefore, women receiving methimazole therapy should be advised against nursing, and reinforces why PTU only should be administered.

Neonatal Graves' Disease

One percent of babies born to women with active Graves' disease can develop hyperthyroidism from the transplacental transfer of maternal TSI.[14] The mother may not necessarily be thyrotoxic. This syndrome can occur in babies born to mothers with Graves' disease whose thyroid glands have already been surgically removed or ablated with ^{131}I, but who exhibit persistently high TSI titers. TSI titers usually fall during pregnancy, and fetal thyroid tissue does not develop until after the twelfth week of gestation. Therefore, TSI measurements in pregnant women with Graves' disease should be deferred until the beginning of the second trimester, to discover which neonates may be at risk for thyrotoxicosis. Maternal TSI titers more than 5 times control values are associated with higher risk. Goiter, tachycardia, accelerated bone age, and craniosynostosis are features of neonatal hyperthyroidism. Thionamide goitrogens can be given to the mother to treat fetal hyperthyroidism in utero, recognized by fetal heart rate and sonogram, even if the mother is euthyroid or hypothyroid, and receiving thyroid replacement therapy. The duration of neonatal hyperthyroidism parallels that of the half-life of the transferred maternal gamma globulin. Therefore, symptoms and signs usually resolve progressively over the first 4 to 8 weeks postpartum.

References

1. Wartofsky L, ed: The thyroid gland. In: Becker KL, ed. *Principles and Practice of Endocrinology and Metabolism*, 2nd ed. Philadelphia, Lippincott, 1995, pp 367-398.

2. Volpé R: Autoimmunity causing thyroid dysfunction. *Endocrinol Metab Clin North Am* 1991;20:565-587.

3. McDougall IR: Graves' disease. Current concepts. *Med Clin North Am* 1991;75:79-95.

4. Rees Smith B, McLachlan SM, Furmaniak J: Autoantibodies to the thyrotropin receptor. *Endocr Rev* 1988;9:106-121.

5. Weetman AP, McGregor AM: Autoimmune thyroid disease: further developments in our understanding. *Endocr Rev* 1994;15:788-830.

6. Bahn RS, Garrity JA, Gorman CA: Diagnosis and management of Graves' ophthalmopathy. Clinical review 13. *J Clin Endocrinol Metab* 1990;71:559-563.

7. Braverman LE, Utiger RD, eds: Werner and Ingbar's *The Thyroid: A Fundamental and Clinical Text*, 7th ed. Philadelphia, Lippincott, 1996, pp 525-558.

8. Aronow WS: The heart and thyroid disease. *Clin Geriatr Med* 1995;11:219-229.

9. Carter JA, Utiger RD: The ophthalmopathy of Graves' disease. *Ann Rev Med* 1992;43:487-495.

10. Franklyn JA: The management of hyperthyroidism. *N Engl J Med* 1994;330:1731-1738.

11. Farrar JJ, Toft AD: Iodine-131 treatment of hyperthyroidism: current issues. *Clin Endocrinol* 1991;35:207-212.

12. Tietgens ST, Leinung MC: Thyroid storm. *Med Clin North Am* 1995;79:169-184.

13. Becks GP, Burrow GN: Thyroid disease and pregnancy. *Med Clin North Am* 1991;75:121-150.

14. McKenzie JM, Zakarija M: Fetal and neonatal hyperthyroidism and hypothyroidism due to maternal TSH receptor antibodies. *Thyroid* 1992;2:155-159.

Chapter 4

Unusual Types of Thyrotoxicosis

In addition to Graves' disease, thyrotoxicosis can develop from numerous other causes, including nodular goiters, subacute thyroiditis, iodine-induced thyrotoxicosis, iatrogenic hyperthyroidism, transient thyrotoxicosis, thyroid carcinoma-induced thyrotoxicosis, TSH-secreting pituitary tumors, thyrotoxicosis caused by placental tumors, and ectopic thyroid tissue-caused thyrotoxicosis (Table 4-1).

Nodular Goiters

The syndrome of thyrotoxicosis with a multinodular goiter occurs most commonly in the elderly and begins slowly. Cardiac symptoms often are present. The syndrome is distinguished from Graves' disease by the absence of eye signs, along with the absence of antibodies to the thyroid-stimulating hormone (TSH) receptor, to thyroglobulin, and to thyroid peroxidase (TPO). On iodine 131 (^{131}I) scan, nodules do not suppress with T_3 administration, and the nonspecific signs of autoimmune activation (eg, relative lymphocytosis, relative neutropenia, splenomegaly) characteristic of Graves' disease, are *absent* in multinodular goiter. Treatment involves ^{131}I administration in dosages larger than those used in Graves' disease. ^{131}I follows pretreatment with antithyroid drugs to normalize circulating thyroid hor-

Table 4-1: Causes of Thyrotoxicosis

- Graves' disease
- Toxic multinodular goiter
- Toxic adenoma
- Subacute thyroiditis
- Postpartum thyrotoxicosis
- TSH-secreting pituitary tumor
- hCG from trophoblastic disease
- Iodide-induced hyperthyroidism
- Thyrotoxicosis factitia
- Ectopic thyroid tissue (struma ovarii)

mone concentrations. This precaution preempts exacerbation of thyrotoxicosis secondary to irradiation-induced thyroiditis in an elderly population at risk for ischemic heart disease.

Single toxic nodules occur infrequently, and are sometimes identified as dominant nodules in multinodular goiter. Single nodules appear most often in young individuals, in contrast to multinodular goiter. Treatment with ^{131}I is ideal because the remainder of the thyroid gland is suppressed by the autonomous hyperfunctioning nodule. Thus, radioiodide is taken up only by the autonomous adenoma.[1] Treatment doses range between 25 and 50 mCi of ^{131}I. A satisfactory alternative to radioiodine is surgical resection of the nodule. Like multinodular goiters, toxic adenomas are not associated with the characteristic autoimmune features of Graves' disease, including exophthalmos. Single nodular hyperactivity has been associated with point mutations in the TSH receptor, which becomes constitutively active in the absence of heightened TSH stimulation.[2]

Subacute Thyroiditis (de Quervain's Thyroiditis)

This syndrome presents as an exquisitely painful enlargement of the thyroid, often with antecedent symptoms of an upper respiratory infection or malaise. Thyrotoxicosis is caused by leaching of thyroid hormones from abnormally permeable thyrocytes. This syndrome is also characterized by fever, arthralgia, asthenia, and anemia. It is classically recognized by an extremely tender thyroid gland, and is associated with a reduced or absent radioactive iodine uptake, suppressed TSH, and a modestly elevated total T_4.[3] The sedimentation rate is usually elevated. Occasionally, only part of the gland may be affected. Because this disease is self-limited, only analgesic medications (eg, nonsteroidal anti-inflammatory drugs [NSAIDs]) or the occasional short-term use of prednisone (30 to 40 mg/d) are required for pain management. There are no permanent sequelae or need for more definitive therapy. Thionamide goitrogens (propylthiouracil [PTU], methimazole [Tapazole®]) are not effective because the thyroid gland does not synthesize excessive thyroid hormones, unlike in Graves' disease.[3] The etiology of this syndrome is not understood, but clusters have been ascribed to the mumps virus, suggesting a viral etiology in some patients. Although fine-needle aspiration biopsy yields a unique and pathognomonic cytology, with characteristic giant cells, biopsy is rarely required. The diagnosis can be established based on the unique clinical features of subacute thyroiditis.

Iodine-Induced Thyrotoxicosis (Jodbasedow)

Excessive iodide administration to individuals with long-standing multinodular goiter can induce thyrotoxicosis that may be quite severe, and persist for months. Because multinodular goiter is characteristically a disorder of the elderly, patients are at risk for thyroid arrhythmias and congestive heart failure. Hyperthyroidism can be precipitated by the administration of iodinated contrast dyes or iodides as expectorants for chronic bronchitis or chronic obstructive pulmonary disease (COPD). If an accurate history of iodine administration cannot be obtained, the diagnosis can be corroborated by the absence of a thyroid uptake, associated with an elevated urinary iodide (collected in an *iodine-free* container). This form of hyperthyroidism can be treated with antithyroid drugs, and, rarely, surgical resection may be necessary.

One source of ^{127}I that is increasing in prevalence is the antiarrhythmic drug amiodarone (Cordarone®), which, in a large series, induced hyperthyroidism in approximately 3% of patients.[4] A dose of 100 mg of amiodarone contains 3 mg of iodine, well above the normal dietary intake in the United States (200 to 600 µg/d). This syndrome can begin from 4 months to 3 years after initiation of amiodarone therapy. The clinical presentation often is dramatic, with recurrence of the original arrhythmias, despite the administration of an antiarrhythmic drug. Thyrotoxicosis should be expected if the heart rate exceeds the pretreatment rate when the arrhythmia recurs, or if the arrhythmia worsens paradoxically during therapy. Other findings include muscle weakness, weight loss, anorexia, restlessness, tremor, diffuse nodular goiter, and congestive heart failure. Because euthyroid patients taking amiodarone often have modestly elevated serum T_4, the diagnosis requires disproportionately greater elevations of T_4 and T_3, usually T_4 concentrations >20 µg/dL or T_3 >200 ng/dL.[4]

Iatrogenic Hyperthyroidism

Hyperthyroidism can be caused by excessive thyroid hormone ingestion, including excessive replacement therapy in hypothyroid patients.[5] It occurs most often in patients ingesting thyroid hormone surreptitiously, particularly by health-care workers, for a variety of reasons, including a desire for weight loss. Thyrotoxicosis in this syndrome is associated with a *small* thyroid gland, an elevation in serum T_4 and T_3 concentrations, and suppressed serum TSH and thyroglobulin. The T_3:T_4 ratio is normal, in contrast to the disproportionate increase in T_3 in thyroid-stimulated states, such as Graves' disease. The ^{131}I thyroid uptake is low to absent. This is a difficult diagnosis to make and often is made by exclusion, because patients usually deny ingestion of thyroid hormones, despite T_4 and T_3 being markedly elevated for no other apparent reason. One epidemic of ingested exogenous thyroxine occurred in the Midwest, attributable to hamburger meat contaminated by thyroid elements in strap muscles from animal sources.

Transient Thyrotoxicosis

Transient thyrotoxicosis (painless or postpartum thyroiditis) most commonly begins after pregnancy (2% to 6% of pregnancies), but a similar process can also occur in men. These patients have small goiters and may have a history of chronic lymphocytic thyroiditis (Hashimoto's disease). Onset characteristically occurs 2 to 5 months after parturition and is moderately severe. The thyrotoxicosis phase may be followed by an interval of euthyroidism and then hypothyroidism for months. Such patients do not have exophthalmos, but often have elevated antibody titers to thyroid peroxidase (TPO) and thyroglobulin (Tg), and the radioactive iodine (RAI) uptake is depressed.[6] No therapy usually is required, but patients may be managed with β-adrenergic blockade or a brief course of corticosteroids during the thyrotoxic phase. Thyroxine replacement is administered to correct the hypothyroidism until completely resolved, which may require up to 12 months.

Thyroid Carcinoma-Induced Thyrotoxicosis

Thyrotoxicosis develops rarely from widespread and metastatic follicular or papillary/follicular thyroid carcinomas. In such individuals, the RAI scan is positive in pulmonary and osseous metastases, serum T_4 and T_3 are elevated, and TSH is suppressed. Hyperthyroidism is treated with ^{131}I therapy, which is also the therapy of choice for eradicating metastases. As in Graves' disease, antithyroid drugs may be used after ^{131}I administration to achieve a euthyroid state before attaining maximum ^{131}I benefit.

TSH-Secreting Pituitary Tumors

Pituitary tumors secreting TSH constitute an uncommon but fascinating cause of hyperthyroidism. They often are initially misdiagnosed as Graves' disease because of the presence of diffuse goiter and signs of thyrotoxicosis. Diagnosis depends on recognition of an inappropriate or elevated serum TSH in the presence of elevated thyroid hormone levels. The serum α subunit of TSH is characteristically disproportionately elevated. However, TSH values can be in the normal range. Patients may require resection of the pituitary tumor, or thyroid ablation with radioiodine. Recent reports, however, describe successful treatment with long-acting somatostatin (Sandostatin®), which inhibits pituitary TSH secretion.[7] About 27% of TSH-secreting tumors also exhibit hypersecretion of other pituitary hormones, including growth hormone (15.7%), prolactin (10.7%), and follicle-stimulating hormone/luteinizing hormone (1.4%).[7]

Hyperthyroidism Associated With Inappropriate Pituitary TSH Secretion

Selective resistance of thyrotrophs to thyroid hormones can lead to mild thyrotoxicosis because the pituitary is less responsive than the periphery to thyroid hormone action. Triiodothyrocetic acid (Triac®) may be useful in controlling this condition.[7] The pathogenesis of this syndrome is not clear, since the TR mutations identified are identical to the syndrome of complete thyroid hormone resistance.

Thyrotoxicosis Caused by Placental Tumors (Choriocarcinoma/Hydatidiform Mole)

Choriocarcinomas and hydatidiform moles can secrete enough human chorionic gonadotropin (hCG), a glycoprotein that possesses approximately 1/10,000 the thyroid-stimulating activity of TSH, to produce mild hyperthyroidism.[8] This syndrome is 10 times as common in the Far East than in the United States, and should be suspected in the *absence* of signs of Graves' disease when an abnormal pregnancy is associated with mild hyperthyroidism, very elevated hCG, and concomitantly suppressed TSH levels. Surgical evacuation of the choriocarcinoma or the hydatidiform mole and chemotherapy eliminate the hyperthyroidism and the trophoblastic malignancy.[9]

Ectopic Thyroid Tissue-Caused Thyrotoxicosis

The presence of hyperfunctioning thyroid tissue in teratomas outside the thyroid bed causing thyrotoxicosis is exceedingly rare. This is exemplified by struma ovarii, in which congenital thyroid elements sometimes occur along with other features (skin and teeth) in the ovary.[10] Therapy is accomplished with surgery, but ^{131}I can be employed if surgery is contraindicated. Some patients have had Graves' disease and strumal thyroid activation, suggesting that circulating thyroid-stimulating immunoglobulin (TSI) stimulated both the normal and abnormal thyroid elements.

References

1. Gorman CA, Robertson JS: Radiation dose in the selection of ^{131}I or surgical treatment for toxic thyroid adenoma. *Ann Intern Med* 1978;89:85-90.

2. Paschke R, Ludgate M: The thyrotropin receptor and thyroid diseases. *N Engl J Med* 1997;337:1675-1681.

3. Greene JN: Subacute thyroiditis. *Am J Med* 1971;51:97-108.

4. Broussolle C, Ducottet X, Martin C, et al: Rapid effectiveness of prednisone and thionamides combined therapy in severe amiodarone iodine-induced thyrotoxicosis. Comparison of two groups of patients with apparently normal thyroid glands. *J Endocrinol Invest* 1989;12:37-42.

5. Ross DS: Subclinical hyperthyroidism: possible danger of overzealous thyroxine replacement therapy. *Mayo Clin Proc* 1988;63:1223-1229.

6. Amino N, Mori H, Iwatani Y, et al: High prevalence of transient post-partum thyrotoxicosis and hypothyroidism. *N Engl J Med* 1982;306:849-852.

7. Beck-Peccoz P, Mariotti S, Guillausseau PJ, et al: Treatment of hyperthyroidism due to inappropriate secretion of thyrotropin with the somatostatin analog SMS-201-995. *J Clin Endocrinol Metab* 1989;68:208-214.

8. Norman RJ, Green-Thompson RW, Jialal I, et al: Hyperthyroidism in gestational trophoblastic neoplasia. *Clin Endocrinol* 1981;15:395-401.

9. Nagataki S, Mizuno M, Sakamoto S, et al: Thyroid function in molar pregnancy. *J Clin Endocrinol Metab* 1977;44:254-263.

10. Piraneo S, Vago L, Gobbi G, et al: Ovarian and cervical thyroid struma. A case report. *Ital J Surg Sci* 1989;19:273-276.

Chapter 5

Hypothyroidism

The constancy of circulating thyroid hormone concentrations is maintained by a dynamic interplay of forces involving hypothalamic thyroid-releasing hormone (TRH), pituitary thyroid-stimulating hormones (TSH), and the thyroid hormones T_4 and T_3. When decompensation occurs in any component of this system, hypothyroidism develops. In its severest form, hypothyroidism is easy to recognize. Typically, however, hypothyroidism is subtle and its recognition more difficult. It is crucial to recognize hypothyroidism because, if left untreated, it can become a chronic, progressive, and potentially lethal process.[1]

Major Manifestations of Hypothyroidism

Most of the major clinical manifestations of overt hypothyroidism can be characterized as a 'slowing down of functions.' This translates into retardation of mental, cardiovascular, GI, and neuromuscular functions. Common symptoms include bradycardia, slow physical movements, slow speech, lethargy, impaired memory, constipation, and intolerance of cold.[2] On physical examination, signs that are relatively specific for hypothyroidism involve the skin and neuromuscular systems, including dry skin, thinning of the lateral eyebrows, and a doughy texture of the dermis. Because hypothyroidism is associated with accumulation of mucopolysaccharides (hyaluronic acid) in the dermis (myxedema), patients often have coarse, cold, skin with facial puffiness and periorbital swelling. Tongue enlargement and vocal hoarseness represent the same process. The ivory-yellow skin of patients with hypothyroidism is caused by carotene accumulation due to impaired carotene conversion to vitamin A. Dry, coarse, and brittle hair is common. The facies often are characteristic, with lack of expressiveness, thickened lips, and drooping upper eyelids, secondary to diminished sympathetic stimulation. The most important neurologic sign is a delay in the relaxation phase of deep tendon reflexes, elicited best when ankle jerks are tested with the patient in a kneeling position on a chair.[1]

Changes in capillary permeability can lead to transudation of fluid across serosal surfaces, including the pericardial, pleural, and peritoneal cavities.

On physical examination, the clinician must determine whether or not the thyroid gland is present and if it is normal size or goitrous.[3]

Etiologies of Hypothyroidism

A knowledge of the etiology of hypothyroidism is required to develop a rational program of management. Most hypothyroidism is a result of dysfunction of the thyroid itself, termed *primary* (or 1°) hypothyroidism (Table 5-1). The most frequently encountered cause of primary hypothyroidism in this country is *idiopathic atrophy*, which occurs more frequently in women than in men, particularly in the fourth decade. In this syndrome, the thyroid gland is atrophic, consisting of fibrous tissue, a few residual thyroid follicles, and lymphocytic and plasma cell infiltration, suggesting the end stages of chronic, autoimmune thyroid disease.[1,2]

Chronic lymphocytic thyroiditis (Hashimoto's thyroiditis) is the second most common cause of primary hypothyroidism, encountered most often in women between the third and sixth decades,[4,5] although it may occur at any age except early childhood. Painless

Table 5-1: Etiology of Hypothyroidism

Primary (high TSH):

- Hashimoto's thyroiditis:
  a. With goiter
  b. Idiopathic thyroid atrophy, presumably end-stage autoimmune thyroid disease, following either Hashimoto's thyroiditis or Graves' disease
- Radioactive iodine therapy for Graves' disease
- Subtotal thyroidectomy for Graves' disease or nodular goiter
- Excessive iodide intake (kelp, radiocontrast dyes)
- Transient thyroiditis
- Rare causes in the USA:
  a. Iodide deficiency
  b. Other goitrogens such as lithium; antithyroid drug therapy
  c. Inborn errors of thyroid hormone synthesis

Secondary (Low TSH, no response to TRH):

- Hypopituitarism due to pituitary adenomas, pituitary ablative therapy, or pituitary destruction

Tertiary (Low TSH, response to TRH):

- Hypothalamic dysfunction (rare) due to tumors or granulomas

Peripheral resistance to the action of thyroid hormone (TR mutations in the ligand-binding domain)

thyromegaly results from cellular infiltration associated with fibrosis and occasionally TSH-mediated hyperplasia. High titers of antibodies to thyroid antigens, including antithyroglobulin and antithyroid peroxidase antibodies (anti-TPO), are identified in more than 90% of such patients.

Another important cause of hypothyroidism is surgical or ^{131}I ablation of the thyroid for the treatment of Graves' disease. After ^{131}I treatment, approximately 20% of patients develop hypothyroidism, with later occurrences at 4%/year. Thus, careful and long-term follow-up of these patients is critically important because most patients will have become hypothyroid by 20 years of age. Interestingly, hypothyroidism may emerge in Graves' patients who have never received surgical or radioiodine ablative therapy, raising the intriguing concept that hypothyroidism may be a late manifestation of the natural history of Graves' disease. Primary hypothyroidism may occur before thyrotoxicosis in Graves' disease, the result of antibodies that block the TSH receptor.

Other causes of primary hypothyroidism are less frequently encountered, including hereditary and environmental determinants. Thyroid dysgenesis is a congenital developmental failure of the thyroid gland, although in most patients small remnants of thyroid tissue in the midline can be demonstrated with isotopic scanning techniques.[6,7]

Genetically determined defects in the biogenesis of thyroid hormones can lead to thyroid deficiency and goiter in infancy and childhood. Abnormalities in iodide transport, I-organification, the synthesis of thyroglobulin, and iodide conservation (dehalogenase defect), have provided insights into how thyroid hormones are normally synthesized in humans.

Finally, primary hypothyroidism can result from environmental goitrogens, including, most importantly, antithyroid drugs (methimazole, PTU), excessive iodide intake in susceptible individuals, and lithium carbonate. Food stuffs in the Cruciferae family, such as cabbage, white turnips, and rutabaga, may induce hypothyroidism in iodide-deficient subjects.

Secondary (also called 2° or pituitary) hypothyroidism is a deficiency of pituitary TSH secretion. In contrast to primary hypothyroidism, secondary hypothyroidism patients always have small, atrophic thyroid glands and tend to have milder symptoms.

Pituitary hypothyroidism is usually caused by pituitary tumors or their surgical removal. Tumors must be distinguished from the pituitary enlargement that may accompany primary hypothyroidism, wherein marked elevations in circulating TSH concentrations are characteristic. In contrast, pituitary-caused hypothyroidism is characterized by TSH usually below normal. Clinical features of 1° and 2° hypothyroidism are qualitatively identical.

Hypothyroidism can also develop from hypothalamic TRH deficiency (tertiary or 3°) hypothyroidism, exemplified by hypothalamic granulomas, CNS tumors, or craniopharyngiomas.

Laboratory Diagnosis of Hypothyroid States

The cardinal laboratory features of all forms of reduced thyroid function, except peripheral resistance, are lowered serum free thyroxine (T_4) concentrations and elevations in circulating TSH (>10 µU/mL).[1,2] Measurement of TSH is clearly the most sensitive test, and patients with only modest elevations in TSH (usually 7 to 10 µU/mL) may appear euthyroid clinically and exhibit normal free T_4 values. These patients represent *subclinical hypothyroidism*, which is compensated through normal regulatory mechanisms. Such patients, however, are at risk to develop overt hypothyroidism and should be followed carefully. In contrast to primary hypothyroidism, serum TSH values are usually not elevated in secondary and tertiary hypothyroidism. However, occasionally TSH values in 3° hypothyroidism are paradoxically elevated, with reduced biological activity. This reflects the effect of TRH not only on the synthesis and secretion of TSH, but also on glycosylation of TSH. Thus, in the absence of TRH, abnormal glycosylation occurs that is associated with a lessened TSH effect.

Measurement of circulating T_3 by RIA, in contrast to T_4, is not recommended in hypothyroidism because T_3 concentrations are frequently normal (approximately 30%) in hypothyroid patients with elevated TSH values. Moreover, T_3 reductions are nonspecific and frequently manifest nonthyroidal states, such as starvation or chronic disease, which impair peripheral conversion of T_4 to T_4. Similarly, thyroidal uptakes with ^{131}I or ^{99}Tc are not useful because normal values frequently overlap the low values of hypothyroidism. Uptakes should be reserved for elucidation of the underlying pathophysiology, exemplified by the high isotopic uptakes found in goitrous patients with iodine deficiency, or the demonstration of rapid dischargibility of ^{131}I after perchlorate administration (Ig) in congenital organification defects of the thyroid.

Other biochemical indices have been developed to reflect the patient's metabolic state. Reductions in sex-steroid binding globulin (SHBG) occur in hypothyroidism. However, elevations of other moieties, including the serum enzymes (SGOT, CPK), serum cholesterol, and β-carotene, and the prolongation of the Achilles reflex relaxation time, should not be used as primary diagnostic tools in hypothyroidism because they lack specificity.

Treatment

Treatment of hypothyroidism with thyroid hormones is one of the most satisfying therapeutic experiences in medicine because the administration of a single, inexpensive, nontoxic and nonallergic molecule (levothyroxine, L-T_4) can result in the complete restoration of normal physiology and complete reversal of symptomatology (Figures 5-1 and 5-2).[7] A number of preparations of thyroid hormones are

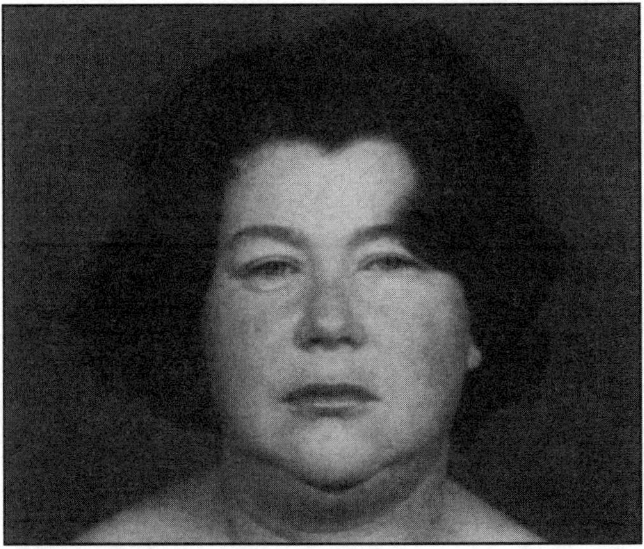

Figure 5-1: Primary hypothyroidism caused by chronic lymphocytic thyroiditis, before treatment. Note facial puffiness, periorbital edema, and dull appearance of the patient's face.

available, and optimal therapy is accomplished with administration of L-T_4, which achieves constant concentrations of both T_4 and T_3, 80% of which is generated from circulating T_4. T_3 itself should not be used because its half-life is brief, and the resultant rapid oscillations in serum concentrations of T_3 from above to below normal may predispose this typically elderly population to supraventricular, life-threatening tachyarrhythmias.[8] Particularly in the elderly, therapy should be initiated with very small dosages of L-T_4 (12.5 to 25 µg p.o. daily), with graded increments at approximately 4-week intervals (25, 50, 75, 100, 112, 125, 150 µg/day) until full replacement is achieved. However, in young, otherwise healthy patients, full replacement therapy can be initiated immediately. Larger L-T_4 dos-

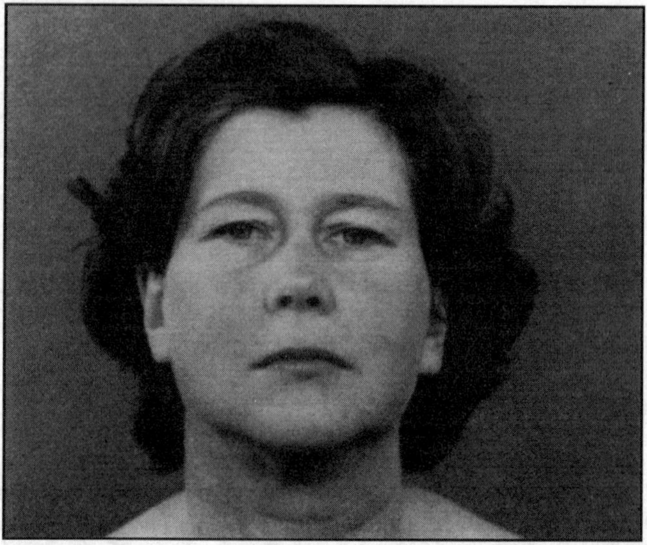

Figure 5-2: Primary hypothyroidism after a 4-month treatment regimen with 0.125 mg of thyroxine PO daily. Note the restoration of an alert appearance, and the absence of facial puffiness and periorbital edema.

ages may be required in selected circumstances, including malabsorption or cirrhosis, and in children. L-T_4 is available in several commercial forms (Synthroid®, Levoxyl®, Levothroid®, Eltroxin®, Levo-T®). The most extensive experience in the largest patient population has been with Synthroid®.

In the elderly, recent evidence suggests that full replacement may be achieved with less L-T_4, about 100 µg/day in patients more than 40 years of age, and occasionally as little as 50 µg/day in those more than 60 years of age. However, because of the large variance in effective dosage at any age, dosage predictions at specific age intervals are imprecise. Consequently, dosage should be individualized. Lower L-T_4 requirements as a function of age have been identified primarily in men. In the elderly, therapy should be undertaken cautiously, with attention to the possibility of precipitating angina pectoris, arrhythmias, myocardial infarction, or CHF, all of which require immediate reductions in L-T_4 dosage.[9]

The primary emphasis of assessment during follow-up should be on *clinical* features, rather than excessive dependency on laboratory determinations. Most signs and symptoms (abnormalities in weight, pulse, reflexes, skin, facies, and the patient's subjective state) disappear gradually within 2 months, with slower resolution in some features (eg, anemia) than in others (weight gain from mucopolysaccharide retention of Na+ and water, serum TSH, and serum cholesterol).

Appropriate laboratory indices include serum free T_4 and TSH, as well as ECGs in the elderly.

Therapy is judged optimal when all symptomatology has been reversed, and when serum FT_4 and serum TSH values are within normal range.[7] TSH should not be suppressed in the treatment of primary hypothyroidism. During pregnancy, L-T_4 requirements rise approximately 30%, and mothers' total (T) T_4 concentrations need to be in the 'pregnancy' range, above nonpartum levels, because of estrogen-induced elevations in TBG binding capacity. Thus, a woman receiving 100 µg/day prepartum may require 150 µg/day intrapartum to raise her TT_4 to 12 to 17 µg/dL, in the pregnancy range.

References

1. Braverman LE, Utiger RD, eds: *Werner and Ingbar's The Thyroid: A Fundamental and Clinical Text*, 7th ed. Philadelphia, Lippincott, 1996, pp 736-883.

2. Wartofsky L, ed: The thyroid gland. In: Becker KL, ed. *Principles and Practice of Endocrinology and Metabolism*, 2nd ed. Philadelphia Lippincott, 1995.

3. Lazarus JH, Hall R, eds: Hypothyroidism and goiter. *Baillieres Clin Endocrinol Metab* 1988;2:531.

4. Volpé R: Autoimmunity causing thyroid dysfunction. *Endocrinol Metab Clin North Am* 1991;20:565-587.

5. Weetman AP, McGregor AM: Autoimmune thyroid disease: further developments in our understanding. *Endocr Rev* 1994;15:788-830.

6. Eckholm R: Biosynthesis of thyroid hormones. *Int Rev Cytol* 1990;120:243.

7. Fisher DA: Clinical review 19. Management of congenital hypothyroidism. *J Clin Endocrinol Metab* 1991;72:523-529.

8. Singer PA, Cooper DS, Levy EG, et al: Treatment guidelines for patients with hyperthyroidism and hypothyroidism. Standards of Care Committee, American Thyroid Association. *JAMA* 1995;273:808-812.

9. Toft AD: Thyroxine therapy. *N Engl J Med* 1994;331:174-180.

Chapter 6

The Euthyroid Sick Syndrome (ESS)

Abnormalities of thyroid function without evidence of thyroid disease occur more commonly than actual disorders of the thyroid (euthyroid sick syndrome, EES). For clinicians, it is extremely important for several reasons to distinguish these abnormalities from thyroid disorders: (1) misinterpretation of a low serum thyroxine (T_4) may lead to inappropriate treatment with thyroid hormones that could be harmful or even lethal, (2) misinterpretation of a high T_4 could lead to iatrogenic hypothyroidism and/or other complications of antithyroid drugs, (3) combined ESS and thyroid disease may preclude making a correct diagnosis of authentic hypothyroidism or hyperthyroidism, interfering with the correct and life-saving treatment in a critically ill patient, and (4), the identification of ESS may provide a useful clue to an unrecognized underlying disease, such as a malignancy.

Classification and Pathophysiology

Thyroid function abnormalities in ESS include: (1) the low triiodothyronine (T_3) syndrome, (2) the low T_3-low T_4 syndrome, (3) high T_4 syndrome, (4) other syndromes. The most common abnormality is a low serum T_3, a finding observed in more than half of all hospitalized patients (Table 6-1).[1] In these patients, mean T_3 values are ap-

Table 6-1: Nonthyroidal Illness Syndromes

- The low T_3 syndrome (the most common)
- The low T_3 and low T_4 syndrome (more severely ill)
- The high T_4 and normal T_3 syndrome (elevated TBG, iopanoic acid, and heparin Rx)

proximately 40% below the normal T_3 concentration. Free T_3 concentrations are also lower, but to a lesser degree. The pathogenesis of the low T_3 state is due primarily to reduced peripheral deiodination of T_4 to T_3 by the enzyme 5' *monodeiodinase*. A wide range of chronic illnesses often reduce this enzyme's biological activity. Serum total T_4 and free T_4 are usually normal in the low T_3 syndrome. Very helpful is the demonstration of an elevated reverse triiodothyronine (rT_3) concentration, in contrast to the low rT_3 in hypothyroidism. The elevated rT_3 in ESS is attributable also to decreased activity of 5' *monodeiodinase*, which also catalyzes the conversion of rT_3 to 3, 3'-diiodothyronine (T_2).

The syndrome of low T_3 and low T_4 is seen in more severely ill patients, often in the intensive care unit, and the finding of a low concentration of serum T4 confers a poor prognosis.[2] In most patients with the low T_4 syndrome, the serum concentration of free T_4, measured by equilibrium dialysis, is usually normal. Interestingly, total T_4 is low even when the serum concentration of its main binding protein, thyroxine-binding globulin (TBG), is normal. The reduction in T_4 in ESS may be caused by the presence of a binding inhibitor, although the nature of this substance has not been completely characterized. One possibility is nonesterified fatty acids derived from damaged tissue. Circulating tissue-derived inhibitors, however, are not found in all patients. Additional pathogenic factors in the low T_4 state include actual reductions in TBG binding capacity, and/or chemical alterations in TBG, such as desialylation, which decreases its affinity for T_4 without altering its affinity for T_3. A third cause of reduced free T_4 concentrations in certain ESS patients is treatment with dopamine or glucocorticoids, which lower circulating TSH. Other factors that may contribute to the low T_4 state are reductions in TSH biological activity, or thyroid resistance to the thyroid actions of TSH.

A third variant of the ESS involves patients who have elevated concentrations of T_4 with normal serum T_3. This commonly results from elevated serum TBG concentrations in chronic liver disorders, including hepatitis and cirrhosis. In these patients, the free T_4 is characteristically normal. A second pathogenetic process in some patients with T_4 elevations involves the action of iodinated radiocontrast agents, such as iopanoic acid. These agents can decrease the hepatic uptake and deiodination of T_4, and can precipitate authentic hyperthyroidism by contributing excess inorganic iodide into autonomous thyroid nodules. Finally, heparin therapy can elevate T_4 concentrations. Heparin is an inhibitor of T_4 binding to TBG. Free T_4 indices is normal in these individuals, however, and they are clinically euthyroid.

There is growing awareness that cytokines may play an important role in the pathogenesis of ESS.[3] Administration of tumor necrosis factor-α or interferon gamma leads to changes in thyroid function that are similar to those found in ESS. TNF-α infusion caused a 36% fall in T_3 and a 48% rise in rT_3. T_4 and free T_4 are not lowered by TNF-α, and Treffer and colleagues have shown that TNF may elevate free T_4 in nonthyroid illness (NTI).

Human immunodeficiency virus (HIV) causes *atypical* changes in thyroid function, including increases in T_4 and TBG, concomitant decreases in rT_3, and the preservation of a normal serum T_3 and T_3/T_4 ratio. Serum T_3, however, may be lowered dramatically in critically ill patients with HIV. The basis for this ESS pattern has not been elucidated.[4]

Evaluation of Thyroid Function in the Presence of ESS

The diagnosis of ESS, particularly when there is concomitant thyroid disease, can be challenging. The most important two measurements are free thyroxine by equilibrium dialysis, and serum TSH by a third-generation assay, to permit detection of values below 0.01 μU/mL.[1] For example, in thyrotoxic patients, serum TSH is usually < 0.01 μU/mL, whereas in ESS syndromes TSH concentrations are 10-fold higher (0.1 μU/mL), except for the lower values found in patients receiving dopamine or glucocorticoids. Conversely, in states of primary hypothyroidism, TSH is usually above 20 μU/mL, whereas elevated TSH values in ESS are usually <15 μU in the vast majority of patients. Subnormal *free* T_4 values in patients receiving dopamine, glucocorticoids, or anticonvulsants suggest true central hypothyroidism. The coexistence of a painless goiter and elevated antibodies to *thyroid peroxidase* strongly favors primary hypothyroidism from chronic lymphocytic thyroiditis (Hashimoto's thyroiditis). The diagnosis of secondary or tertiary hypothyroidism may require additional investigation because serum TSH concentrations can be *normal*, paradoxically elevated, or low. In ESS patients, plasma cortisol, prolactin, and gonadotropins are typically normal, so that the demonstration of a subnormal plasma cortisol and/or low gonadotropin levels, with an elevated prolactin, would favor a central cause for hypothyroidism. Finally, because of these difficulties in interpretation, evaluation of pituitary and thyroid functions should be deferred until enough time has passed to allow for full recovery from ESS, about 2 to 3 weeks.

Therapy for ESS

Most patients with ESS are euthyroid, as reflected by normal free T_3 and free T_4 concentrations, and do not require treatment. However, patients with prolonged illness and with low free T_4 concentrations may be authentically hypothyroid. Whether or not to treat these individuals remains controversial, and most studies that have examined thyroid hormone administration in ESS have not shown benefit.[2] Although this may be due in part to impaired 5' monodeiodination of T_4 to T_3, studies evaluating the administration of T_3 itself in these patients have revealed no clear therapeutic effects either. The one setting in which T_3 treatment has been found to be useful is in patients undergoing open heart surgery. In these procedures, the administration of T_3 acutely has restored aerobic metabolism to an ischemic myocardium and has exerted other favorable influences on cardiac status. Clearly, more studies are needed to clarify which patient populations can possibly benefit from treatment and to determine potential untoward effects of T_4 and/or T_3 therapy in these settings. At this time, T_4 or T_3 therapy should be withheld from ESS patients except in the rare patient with low free thyroid hormone concentrations in whom thyroid hormone therapy may offer some therapeutic advantages without significant risk.

References

1. Lazarus JH, Hall R, eds: Hypothyroidism and goiter. *Baillieres Clin Endocrinol Metab* 1988;2:531.

2. McIver B, Gorman CA: Euthyroid sick syndrome: an overview. *Thyroid* 1997;7:125-132.

3. Bartalena L, Brogioni S, Grasso L, et al: Relationship of the increased serum interleukin-6 concentration to changes of thyroid function in nonthyroidal illness. *J Endocrinol Invest* 1994;17:269-274.

4. Lo Presti JS, Fried JC, Spencer CA, et al: Unique alternations of thyroid hormone indices in the acquired immunodeficiency syndrome (AIDS). *Ann Intern Med* 1989;110:970-975.

Chapter 7

Thyroiditis Syndromes: Acute, Subacute, Chronic Thyroiditis (Autoimmune and Riedel's Struma)

Several important thyroid syndromes are associated with human autoimmunity. Chronic lymphocytic thyroiditis (Hashimoto's disease) is the most common, but closely related diseases are postpartum thyroiditis, idiopathic myxedema with thyroid atrophy and fibrosis, Riedel's struma, and Graves' disease.[1]

The possible role of autoimmune mechanisms as a cause of thyroid disease was first suggested in the mid-1950s by Rose and Witebsky, who produced experimental thyroiditis in rabbits immunized against their own thyroid as an extract suspended in Freund's adjuvant. The presence of precipitating antibodies to thyroglobulin was then demonstrated in patients with thyroiditis, and the recognition of the Long-Acting Thyroid Stimulator (LATS), now called TSI, in the serum of Graves' disease was demonstrated by Adams and Purves in New Zealand. Three thyroidal antigens are particularly important: thyroglobulin (Tg), thyroid peroxidase (anti-TPO), and the thyroid-stimulating hormone (TSH) receptor itself. Other antigens may be involved in thyroid orbitopathy, including the iodide symporter and a 64 kb protein in the orbit.

Hashimoto's Disease

Chronic lymphocytic thyroiditis is one of the most common immunologic disorders in the endocrine system and is associated with chronic hypothyroidism in most cases. It typically presents as a painless, diffuse goiter with local lymphadenopathy, which must be distinguished from thyroid cancers or lymphoma. More than 80% of patients with chronic lymphocytic thyroiditis have thyroid autoantibodies, most importantly anti-TPO, that are very helpful in confirming the diagnosis. Hashimoto's disease occurs in genetically susceptible populations because specific genetic markers have been associated with the development of this disease.[2] However, because the vast majority of individuals who have these markers are normal, other factors must be involved, including the environment. Thyroiditis, for example, can develop after viral infections, suggesting that nonspecific inflammation can initiate a specific immune response in the thyroid gland. Pathologic examination of the thyroid with chronic lymphocytic thyroiditis shows marked destruction of thyroid follicles and extensive infiltration of lymphoid cells. These cells often form terminal centers in or around thyroid follicular cells. The result of this inflammatory process is destruction of thyroid follicular cells and eventual hypofunction of the thyroid gland.

Pathogenesis

The pathogenesis of lymphocytic thyroiditis appears to involve an initiating inflammatory event, such as a viral infection, followed by a specific autoreactive response from the immune system. A number of viruses have been postulated to induce autoimmunity in the thyroid gland, including human T-cell lymphotrophic virus type I.[3] Viral infection not only stimulates antibody production, but also generates a number of important cytokines, including interleukins (IL) 1β, IL-2, IL-4, IL-6, IL-8, and IL-10. There is an influx of T cells reactive to thyroid antigens. The T cells involved in this response appear restricted in the use of antigen receptor β-chain genes, indicating genetic determinants. The actual mechanism of thyroid cell destruction is not completely understood, but an important process involves cytotoxic T cell lysis of thyroid follicular cells, probably through the Fas pathway, since the Fas ligand can cause activation of apoptosis in thyroid follicular cells.[3] Antibody-dependent cellular cytotoxicity has also been suggested as having a role in thyroid follicular cell destruction, although supporting data are scant. Thyroid dysfunction may result from the loss of intracellular matrix molecules, such as integrins. The loss of matrix structure interferes with thyrocyte communication to affect the coordinated development of thyroid follicles and the production of thyroid hormone, a process that leads to hypothyroidism. Antibodies to Tg and TPO are key markers of this disease and may also participate in antibody-dependent cytotoxicity.

Occasionally, patients with Hashimoto's thyroiditis may also develop Graves' disease, including ophthalmopathy or pretibial myxedema. Investigators speculate that these patients initially develop thyroiditis and hypothyroidism with antibodies blocking the TSH receptor response to endogenous TSH. Later, the spectrum of circulating antibodies is altered to contain TSI, which activates the TSH receptor, like pituitary TSH.

Diagnosis and Treatment

Hashimoto's thyroiditis is usually easy to recognize (Table 7-1). Patients present with a painless goiter with either euthyroidism or mild clinical hypothyroidism. By a 4-to-1 ratio, it is more common in women than in men. Patients are often unaware of their thyroid enlargement. The thyroid gland is usually firmer than normal, in contrast to the softer texture of the vascular thyroid gland in Graves' disease. Older patients with hypothyroidism have a small, firm, atrophic thyroid gland, sug-

Table 7-1: Signs and Symptoms of Hashimoto's Disease

- painless diffuse goiter
- more common in women than men (4:1 ratio)
- thyroid gland firmer than normal
- TSH may be elevated
- low circulating T_4 may be present
- autoantibodies, particularly anti-Tg and anti-TPO, are elevated
- large number of lymphocytes, plasma cells, and sometimes Hürthle cells on fine-needle aspiration

gesting the possibility of burned-out earlier lymphocytic thyroiditis. The diagnosis can be corroborated by demonstrating an elevated TSH, a low circulating free thyroxine (T_4), and elevations of autoantibodies, particularly to Tg and TPO. Occasionally, fine-needle biopsy of the gland is useful, particularly if the clinical syndrome is associated with nodularity of the thyroid gland or a predominant nodule, which needs to be distinguished from a benign or malignant neoplasm. The fine-needle aspirate in Hashimoto's will demonstrate large numbers of lymphocytes and the presence of Hürthle cells (Figure 7-1).

Because 10% to 15% of young patients presenting with goiter in hypothyroidism progress to permanent hypothyroidism, clinicians must recognize this syndrome and initiate appropriate therapy. The indications for treatment are similar to those described above for hypothyroidism, and the patient should be rendered euthyroid with T_4 orally, without the use of triiodothyronine (T_3). Surgical removal of the thyroid is rarely indicated because goiters are small

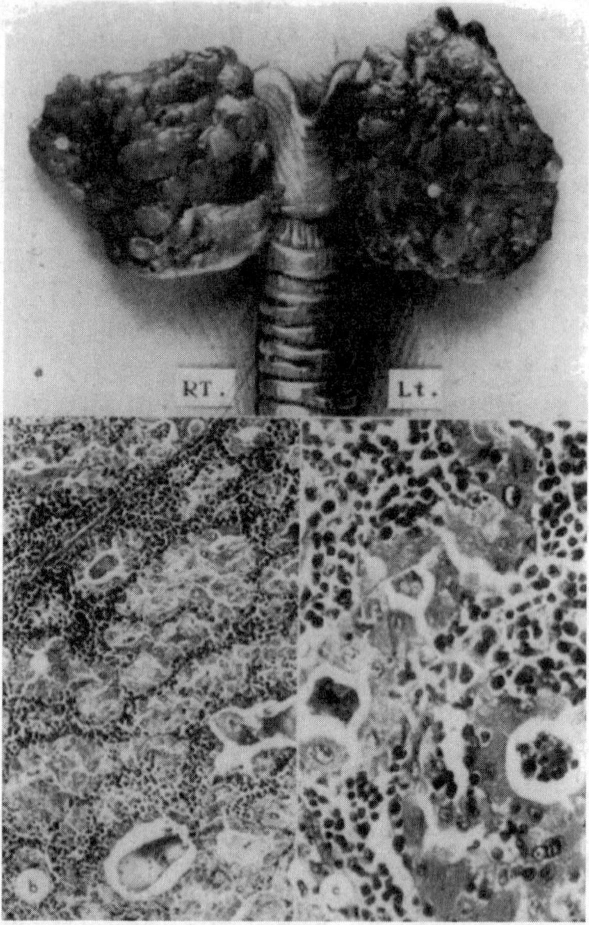

Figure 7-1: Hashimoto's thyroiditis. A, the lobular pattern of the thyroid grossly. B, interfollicular infiltration by lymphocytes and plasma cells. C, granular oxyphylic changes in the cytoplasm of the follicular epithelium (Askanazy cells). From Woolner LB, et al: *J Clin Endocrinol Metab* 1959;19:53-83.

and do not cause any impairment of function of the airway, esophagus, or recurrent laryngeal nerves.

Because Hashimoto's thyroiditis may be part of a syndrome of autoimmune, polyglandular deficiency, patients must be monitored for pernicious anemia, adrenal insufficiency, and diabetes mellitus, in addition to hypothyroidism.

Other Forms of Thyroiditis

The four other forms of thyroiditis (Table 7-2) are acute thyroiditis, subacute thyroiditis (de Quervain's), postpartum thyroiditis, and granulomatous thyroiditis (Riedel's struma). Acute thyroiditis represents infection in the thyroid gland in the context of a systemic infection. Patients are usually quite ill and febrile. Metastatic bacterial or fungal abscesses are encountered in the thyroid and can be confirmed by aspiration. This diagnosis should be suspected in immunocompromised hosts, such as patients with AIDS. It does not lead to any acute or chronic impairment in thyroid function. Importantly, clinicians must differentiate a mass lesion of the thyroid as an abscess, instead of an adenoma or carcinoma. Therapy entails appropriate antimicrobials and surgical drainage, if appropriate.

Subacute thyroiditis is a unique inflammatory disorder of the thyroid gland, probably caused by viral infections.[4] A number of viruses have been implicated, including Coxsackie, mumps, and adenoviruses. Antibody titers to viruses often rise acutely. Although biopsy is rarely needed to make this diagnosis, pathologic examination reveals thyroid enlargement with unique, pathognomic giant cells in and around thyroid follicles (Figure 7-2).

Subacute thyroiditis presents with antecedent malaise, fever, and exquisite tenderness to palpation of the thyroid gland. This unique degree of tenderness is virtually diagnostic. There is no ophthalmopathy or pretibial myxedema, but patients may display mild thyrotoxicosis caused by

Table 7-2: Four Types of Thyroiditis Syndromes

Type of Thyroiditis	Thyroid Status
Acute	Euthyroid
Subacute	Mildly thyrotoxic
Chronic	Euthyroid, or hypothyroid, rarely hyperthyroid
Riedel's struma	May become hypothyroid

increased permeability of damaged thyroid cells. Laboratory findings include elevations in free T_4 and free T_3, low TSH, and extremely low or absent radioactive iodine uptake. A helpful laboratory determination is the sedimentation rate, which is invariably elevated. Importantly, thyroid autoantibodies, in contrast to lymphocytic thyroiditis, are *not* elevated.

The course of this disease is such that spontaneous resolution will ultimately occur without permanent hypothyroidism or hyperthyroidism. Resolution occurs over weeks or months, and the patient should be treated symptomatically with acetaminophen or NSAIDs. Occasionally, a short course of corticosteroids (eg, prednisone, 40 mg/day for several weeks) can be administered to reduce in-

Pathology	Course
Bacterial abscess formation—fluctuant texture	Abscess surgically drained and antimicrobials resolve the inflammation.
Langhan's giant cells. Texture normal but exquisite tenderness.	Spontaneous resolution. No sequelae.
Lymphocytic and infiltration, and Askanazy cells Thyroid texture firmer than normal.	Gradual loss of normal function may occur secondary to cell necrosis by lymphocytes.
Dense fibrosis, extension to outside structures. Thyroid texture is 'stony' hard.	Progressive loss of thyroid function and possible extrinsic compression of trachea and/or esophagus.

tense pain not relieved with analgesics. Antithyroid drugs (PTU, Tapazole®) are ineffectual and therefore should not be used.

Postpartum Thyroiditis

Postpartum thyroiditis presents characteristically with mild and transient thyrotoxicosis, and a low radioactive iodide uptake beginning at 2 to 6 months after delivery.[5] Hyperthyroidism is often followed by a longer period of hypothyroidism, lasting several months to even a year. Ultimately, all features are resolved spontaneously. The clinical presentation may include thyrotoxicosis alone (50%), hypothyroidism alone (25%), or both phases sequentially (25%) (Figure 7-3).

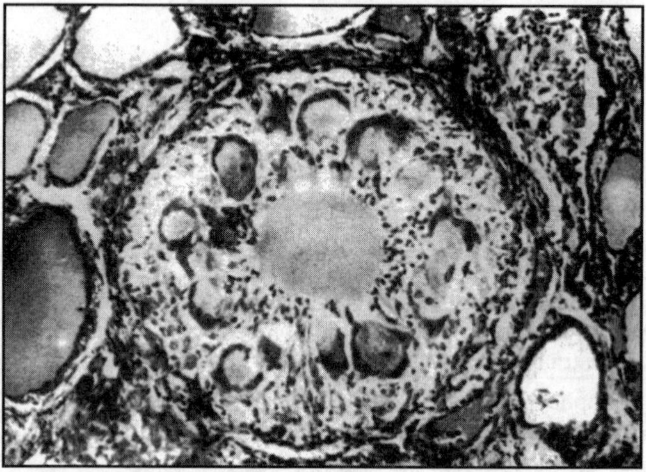

Figure 7-2: Subacute thyroiditis. An intrafollicular giant cell surrounding a central core of colloid, its unique histopathology. From Meachim G, Young MH: J *Clin Patho*l 1963;16:189-199.

Postpartum thyroiditis occurs in approximately 10% of pregnancies; and, importantly, in more than 30% in women with positive anti-TPO antibodies. Postpartum thyroiditis is strongly associated with HLA-DR3 and HLA-DR5 haplotypes, known to be associated also with chronic lymphocytic thyroiditis. The activation of thyroiditis after parturition probably represents a resurgence of the autoimmune process after its suppression during the intrapartum period. Thyroid function should be evaluated by measuring free thyroxine (FT_4) and TSH levels in women during the postpartum period who have had evaluations in serum TPO Ab, and in all women with possible symptoms of thyroid dysfunction, ascribed erroneously to postpartum depression or other psychological factors.

Treatment of the hyperthyroid phase is symptomatic, with β-blockers. Antithyroid drugs are ineffective, because

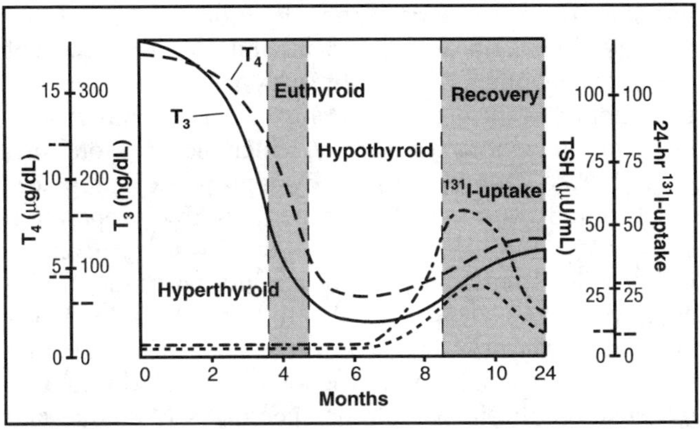

Figure 7-3: The triphasic clinical pattern of postpartum thyroiditis. Note the initial hyperthyroid phase, followed by a brief euthyroid interval, and a longer hypothyroid phase, which then undergoes complete resolution. From Woolf ED: *Endocrine Rev* 1980;1: 411-420.

the thyrotoxicosis is caused by altered permeability of thyrocytes and not by stimulated secretion from the thyroid gland, as in Graves' disease. During the hypothyroid phase, patients usually require thyroid hormone replacement, which should be discontinued when this phase is completed. Therapy with oral thyroxine might be needed for many months (>12).

Transient thyroiditis can occur also in women who are not pregnant, and in males at a lower prevalence.

Riedel's Struma

Chronic granulomatous thyroiditis, or Riedel's struma, presents clinically with an extremely firm to rock-like thyroid gland.[6] Extension is common outside the thyroid into overlapping muscular and surrounding soft tissues, and occasionally into the retroperitoneum. The hardness of the thyroid gland requires clinicians to differentiate it from papillary or follicular carcinoma by biopsy. The histopathology reveals fibrosis and eosinophilia. Compromise of the tracheal lumen, encroachment on the esophagus, or interruption of the recurrent laryngeal nerves with hoarseness, are indications for therapy, which includes total surgical thyroidectomy, followed by appropriate T_4 replacement therapy with an appropriate thyroxine preparation such as Synthroid®, Levoxyl®, Levothroid®, Eltroxin®, or Levo-T®. Riedel's struma occurs primarily in middle-aged women, and low titers of anti-Tg and anti-TPO may be present. The etiology, however, is unclear. Although it may be a variant of lymphocytic thyroiditis (Hashimoto's), the eosinophilia in pathologic specimens is unique and not encountered usually in Hashimoto's disease or in its transient variants.

References

1. Amino N: Autoimmunity and hypothyroidism. *Baillieres Clin Endocrinol Metab* 1988;2:591-617.

2. Nagataki S, Mori T, Torizuma K: 80 years of Hashimoto's disease. *Excerpta Medica* 1993; International Congress Series 1028.

3. Baker JR Jr: Autoimmune endocrine disease. *JAMA* 1997;278: 1931-1937.

4. Volpé R: The management of subacute (de Quervain's) thyroiditis. *Thyroid* 1993;3:253-255.

5. Amino N, Mori H, Iwatani Y, et al: High prevalence of transient postpartum thyrotoxicosis and hypothyroidism. *N Engl J Med* 1982;306:849-852.

6. Chopra D, Wool MS, Crosson A, et al: Riedel's struma associated with subacute thyroiditis, hypothyroidism and hypoparathyroidism. *J Clin Endocrinol Metab* 1978;46:869-871.

Chapter 8

Thyroid Enlargement: Diffuse and Nodular Goiters

Thyroid nodules are common and must be investigated to rule out thyroid malignancies. Nodules can be single or multiple, nonpalpable or palpable. Importantly, nodule prevalence increases after exposure to ionizing radiation and when a diet is deficient of iodine. New nodules are about 6 times more frequent in women than in men, while thyroid cancer is only slightly more prevalent in women than men. Therefore, the likelihood of a nodule being malignant is much lower in female patients than in male counterparts. In the Framingham study, thyroid nodules have been reported in 6.4% of women and 1.5% of men between 30 and 59 years of age. With an incidence of about 0.1% a year, an estimated 250,000 new thyroid nodules will occur in the United States this year.[1]

Clinical Assessment

Most nodules present as an asymptomatic, painless thyroid mass, discovered by the physician or occasionally the patient. Relevant history includes prior exposure to irradiation, particularly for childhood tonsillar enlargement or status thymus lymphaticus.[2] Nodules are more common in younger patients (less than 20 years) than in older

Table 8-1: Features Suggesting Malignant Thyroid Nodules
Sex: More prevalent in men
Age: More common in younger patients (<20 years)
Vocal cord involvement: Hoarseness
Extension: Tumor growth by local extension
Radiation exposure: Prior exposure increases risk.

patients (more than 60 years). A helpful mnemonic regarding the malignancy potential of any given nodule is SAVER, an acronym for Sex, Age, Vocal cord involvement, Extension, and Radiation exposure (Table 8-1). Physical findings that suggest, but are not necessarily diagnostic, of carcinoma include very firm or hard nodules, fixation to adjacent structures, vocal cord paralysis, and the presence of lymphadenopathy. Common etiologies of thyroid nodules include follicular and Hürthle cell adenomas, benign cysts, papillary or follicular carcinomas, and, occasionally, nodular Hashimoto's thyroiditis. Uncommon causes of nodules are infection, medullary carcinoma, anaplastic carcinoma, lymphoma, and metastatic cancer from another site.

Fine-Needle Aspiration Biopsy

In the past, the standard evaluation of nodules included initial thyroid scans and/or thyroid ultrasound examinations. Now, however, a fine-needle aspiration biopsy (FNA) is the best initial step toward defining the nature of a thyroid nodule. FNA is performed in an ambulatory setting. Fine-needle aspiration biopsy is about 95% accurate, 92% specific, and 83% sensitive, with a 5% false-negative rate.[3] FNA is safe and has essentially no complications.

FNA Technique

To perform this procedure, the following supplies are needed: an aspiration 'gun' (Cameco Syringe, Precision Dynamics Corporation, Burbank, CA), a 20 cc disposable plastic syringe, appropriate needles (23-25 bore), clean glass slides with frosted ends, a pencil for labeling slides, a Copeland jar with 95% alcohol, a slide box for air-dried smears, Saccomanno's fixative in a clear jar for rinsing needles and/or tissue fragments, and a pair of gloves.[4] All slides should be lined up and labeled before FNA is performed. Up to three pairs of slides are prepared from each aspiration, and each slide pair should consist of one air-dried and one smear fixed in 95% alcohol. We recommend performing at least 4 separate aspirations. The aspiration pistol is held in one hand while the second and third fingers of the other hand immobilize the thyroid nodule to ensure entry of the needle into the nodule. When it is necessary to biopsy a *nonpalpable nodule* (visualized by ultrasound), aspiration should be performed under ultrasonic guidance. If the aspiration yields cystic fluid, expel 1 to 2 drops of the fluid onto 3 slides and prepare 3 slide pairs as described above. After the smears are prepared, the rest of the fluid should be placed in the Saccomanno's fixative. For cyst fluid characterization, record the amount as well as the color of the aspirated fluid. Crystal-clear fluid raises the rare possibility of parathyroid origin, and high parathyroid hormone levels in the aspirated fluid confirm this diagnosis.[4]

Cytologies are reported as satisfactory or diagnostic in 85% of specimens, and nondiagnostic in the remainder. The most common benign, or negative, cytodiagnosis is a colloid or benign thyroid nodule. These cytological examinations usually show abundant cytoplasm and normal epithelial cells. Other nonmalignant diagnoses include cystic lesions, lymphocytic thyroiditis, and subacute, or granulomatous, thyroiditis. Papillary carcinomas account for 70% to 80% of malignant lesions and can usually be diagnosed confidently by FNA. Papillary carcinoma biopsies yield cytologies with large nuclei and irregular shapes. The field is hypercellular and papillary in configuration. There is pale chromatin, dense cytoplasm, and absent colloid. The problematic group includes *follicular neoplasms*, Hürthle cell neoplasms, and specimens with cellular atypia. Benign follicular neoplasms *cannot* be separated from follicular carcinomas by the absence of capsular invasion or entry into lymph nodes or other metastatic foci. These follicular neoplasms are hypercellular with cells arranged in micro follicular patterns. Aspirates with adequate epithelial cells in this nondiagnostic category account for 15% to 20% of specimens.

Criteria for judging adequacy of aspirates is arbitrary. It is helpful to have the cytologist present at the biopsy to examine specimens for adequacy of cellularity before completing the FNA. We feel that a satisfactory smear should contain at least five groups of cells, each group consisting of at least 10 to 12 cells. In a large series performed on 15,210 biopsies at the Mayo Clinic, 64% were negative, 11% were suspicious, 4% were positive, and 21% were nondiagnostic. Thus, a diagnosis could be made on about 80% of the aspirates. If there is more than one nodule, other nodules may need to be aspirated also, even if there is a dominant nodule present. For the patient concerned about discomfort of the biopsy procedure, which is minimal, applying an ice cube to the skin for a few moments will provide adequate analgesia without the need to use local anesthesia by intradermal injection, which can be more uncomfortable than the subsequent aspiration itself.[5]

Therapy of Thyroid Nodules

Most nodules are managed by follow-up visits, FNA (where appropriate), and/or suppression with L-thyroxine. The use of T_4 for nodular suppression has become questioned, and many newer studies indicate that the response rate to suppression is quite low, about 20%.[6] We do not recommend thyroid hormone suppression in the routine management of thyroid nodules. Moreover, spontaneous regression of nodules occurs in about half of patients, making the interpretation of nodular involution difficult. In addition, thyroid carcinomas under TSH stimulation may also shrink on T_4 therapy, and clinicians cannot assume that a nodule is benign on the basis of regression after thyroid hormone therapy. In the elderly, long-term suppression therapy with T_4 can lead to subclinical osteopenia and/or atrial cardiac arrhythmias, particularly atrial fibrillation.

Nodular goiters that have more than one palpable nodule require a more complex scheme of management.[7] To exclude malignancy in these patients, biopsies may be required from multiple nodules. Imaging with CT or MRI may be helpful in determining the size of a multinodular goiter, the number of nodules, and whether there is substernal extension. It is critical to perform an FNA on: (1) a dominant nodule, (2) a growing nodule, and (3) fixed nodules. Nodules judged by biopsy or clinical criteria to be suspicious for malignancy should be removed surgically.[4]

In patients with benign, multinodular goiters, annual evaluation is appropriate. Patients who are thyrotoxic or have local compression symptoms involving airway or esophagus, or even those patients desiring resection for cosmetic considerations, should be referred for surgical management.

In the euthyroid asymptomatic patient, medical management is usually sufficient for multinodular goiters. In selected circumstances, patients with very large multinodular goiters, with normal thyroid function tests or suppressed TSH level without clinical thyrotoxicosis, may benefit from radioiodine or surgery. To accomplish adequate radioiodine uptake by these nodules, it is useful to lower the extracellular iodide pool with diuretics and prescribe a low iodine diet, followed by a higher-than-usual dose of ^{131}I than that used for the treatment of Graves' disease. The choice of therapy depends on the patient's medical condition, the radioiodine uptake, and the availability of suitable surgical skills for thyroid resection. The preferred approach to solitary toxic nodules, which account for about 5% of all nodules, is ^{131}I therapy. Because the rest of the thyroid gland is suppressed, only the hyperfunctioning nodule takes up the ^{131}I, so the remainder of the thyroid bed is protected. Surgery, however, is an excellent alternate choice to manage single, hyperfunctioning nodules. We do not recommend therapy with ethanol injection into toxic nodules under sonographic guidance because of the risks of hematoma and vocal cord paralysis, or in some cases, thyroidal dysplasia.[8]

Nonpalpable Nodules

Sensitive imaging techniques can now reveal nonpalpable thyroid nodules, which pose a management problem. Clearly, such nodules must be evaluated identically to those that are palpable, and not simply disregarded as incidentalomas. Therefore, FNA biopsy during ultrasound guidance is the diagnostic test that should be performed to evaluate the malignant potential of these lesions.[9]

In summary, the strategy of using FNA as the first diagnostic probe in all circumstances, excepting nonpalpable nodules, has become established as safe and cost-effective; also, FNA often prevents inappropriate surgery in patients. The routine use of T_4 for suppression is no longer recommended because it is not effective and may be harmful.

References

1. Mazzaferri EL, de los Santos ET, Rofagha-Keyhani S: Solitary thyroid nodule: diagnosis and management. *Med Clin North Am* 1988;72:1177.

2. Rojeski MT, Gharib H: Nodular thyroid disease: evaluation and management. *N Engl J Med* 1985;313:428.

3. Gharib H, Goellner JR: Fine-needle aspiration biopsy of the thyroid: an appraisal. *Ann Intern Med* 1993;118:282-289.

4. Gharib H: Changing concepts in the diagnosis and management of thyroid nodules. *Endocrinol Metab Clin North Am* 1997;26:777-800.

5. Oertel YC: Fine-needle aspiration and the diagnosis of thyroid cancer. *Endocrinol Metab Clin North Am* 1996;25:69-91.

6. Ridgway EC: Clinical review 30: clinician's evaluation of a solitary thyroid nodule. *J Clin Endocrinol Metab* 1992;74:231-235.

7. Tan GH, Gharib H, Reading CC: Solitary thyroid nodule. Comparison between palpation and ultrasonography. *Arch Intern Med* 1995;155:2418-2423.

8. Lippi F, Ferrari C, Manetti L, et al: Treatment of solitary autonomous thyroid nodules by percutaneous ethanol injection: results of an Italian multicenter study. The Multicenter Study Group. *J Clin Endocrinol Metab* 1996;81:3261-3264.

9. Tan GH, Gharib H: Thyroid incidentalomas: management approaches to nonpalpable nodules discovered incidentally on thyroid imaging. *Ann Intern Med* 1997;126:226-231.

Chapter 9

Thyroid Imaging: Indications and Interpretations

Imaging of the thyroid gland provides information about the size, shape, and distribution of functional activity of the thyroid gland. Imaging is primarily used to assess single or multiple nodules. Scans are rarely indicated in Graves' disease, where there is diffused hyperplasia of the thyroid gland. Two isotopes are routinely used for thyroid imaging, ^{123}I and ^{99}Tc 99m pertechnetate. ^{123}I is administered orally but scans of the thyroid cannot be performed until 24 hours (Figure 9-1), whereas ^{99}Tc is administered intravenously and scans can be obtained within 1 hour.[1] Thyroid images from these radioisotopes are achieved with either a gamma camera or a rectilinear scanner that moves back and forth across the target area, giving a life-size image of the thyroid. The gamma camera is equipped with a pinhole collimator, which yields images with higher sensitivity, specificity, overall accuracy, and more rapid imaging time.

Imaging Thyroid Nodules

When the radiodensity of a nodule is greater than the surrounding thyroid, it is considered a 'hot nodule.'[2] Nodules that have lesser density than the surrounding normal tissue are termed 'cold nodules.'[2] The incidence

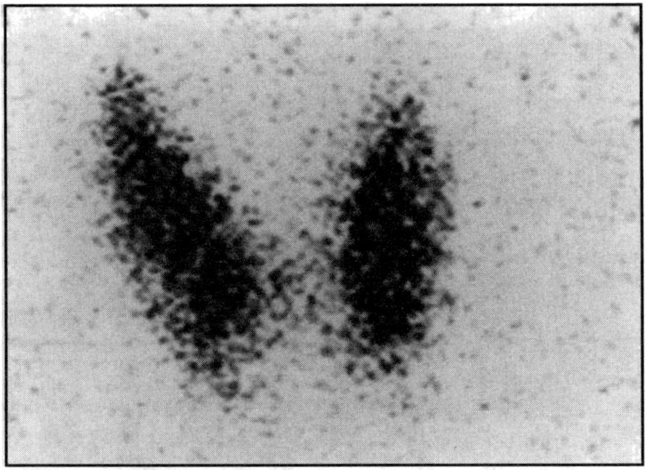

Figure 9-1: Image of the normal thyroid gland made 6 hours after an oral dose of 200 mCi of ^{123}I. Note that the lobes are symmetrical and that the isthmus is not well visualized. Serum free thyroxine and TSH levels were normal. (Used with permission, from: Braverman LE, Utger RD, eds. *The Thyroid Gland.* Philadelphia, Lippincott-Raven, 1991).

of cancer in hot nodules (Figure 9-2), which are sufficiently functional to suppress the remaining thyroid gland, is vanishingly small. However, about 15% of cold nodules have been shown to be malignant. When it is necessary to visualize thyroid tissue under the sternum, such as goiters that have extended inferiorly, or to visualize potential metastases from thyroid cancer in bone or lung, ^{131}I is the isotope of choice because of its longer half-life and higher radioactive emission energy.

The radiopharmaceutical of choice for routine nodule screening is Tc 99m pertechnetate. Although ^{123}Iodine can produce suitable images, results with ^{123}I do not provide more useful information than that attained with Tc 99m

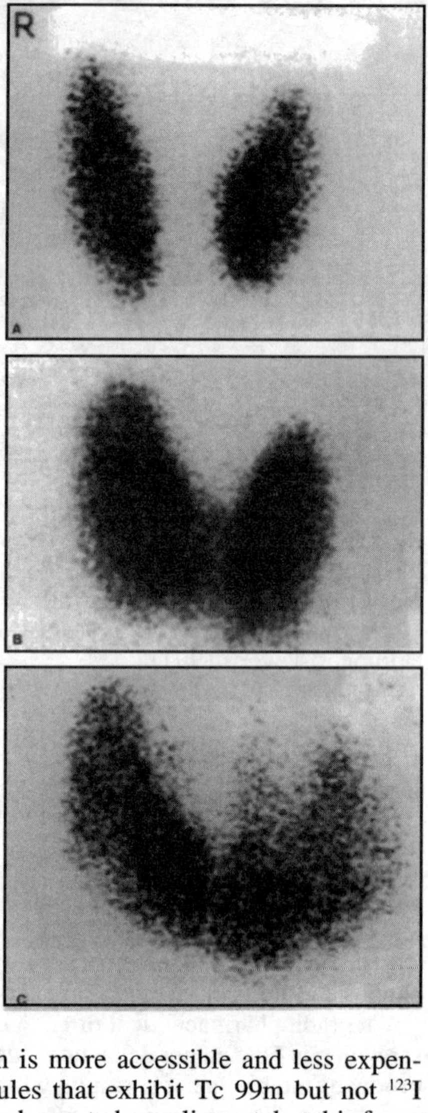

Figure 9-2: Thyroid scintiscans from 3 patients with Graves' disease and hyperthyroidism. Note the enlargement of thyroid lobes (A-C), the imaged isthmus (B,C), and there is virtually no background. The pyramidal lobe (C) arises from the medial aspect of the left lobe. In all 3 patients, the thyroid uptake was considerably elevated, between 60% and 80%. (Used with permission, from: Braverman LE, Utger RD, eds. *The Thyroid Gland*. Philadelphia, Lippincott-Raven, 1991).

(Figure 9-2), which is more accessible and less expensive. The rare nodules that exhibit Tc 99m but not ^{123}I retention have been shown to be malignant, but this func-

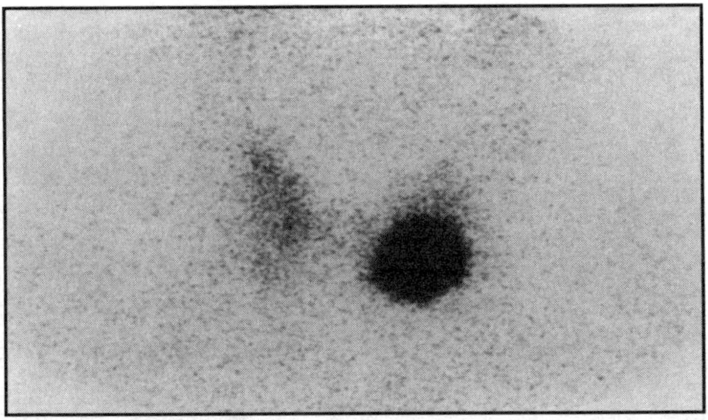

Figure 9-3: Image of a thyroid gland with a palpable, hyperfunctioning nodule in the left lobe, made with ^{99}Tc 99m pertechnetate. The function in the remainder of the thyroid gland is suppressed. (Used with permission, from: Sason JC: Selection of the optimal scanning agent for thyroid cancer. In: *Thyroid* 1997, pp 295-302).

tional dissociation is uncommon, and its identification does not justify routine images with both isotopes.[2]

Imaging Papillary and Follicular Thyroid Carcinomas

The purpose of thyroid imaging in patients with documented thyroid cancer is to identify and localize potential metastatic tissue, or residual thyroid bed carcinoma tissue, to develop rational treatment for optimal outcome.[3] Until recently, all, or nearly all, of the normal thyroid tissue had to be removed to generate TSH elevations of sufficient magnitude (25 to 50 mU/L) to permit visualization of functioning thyroid malignant tissues. Recombinant human TSH (rhTSH, Thyrogen®) has now become available and eliminates the need to discontinue T_4 and/or T_3 for both total body scanning and quantification of circulating thyroglobulin with and without TSH stimulation.

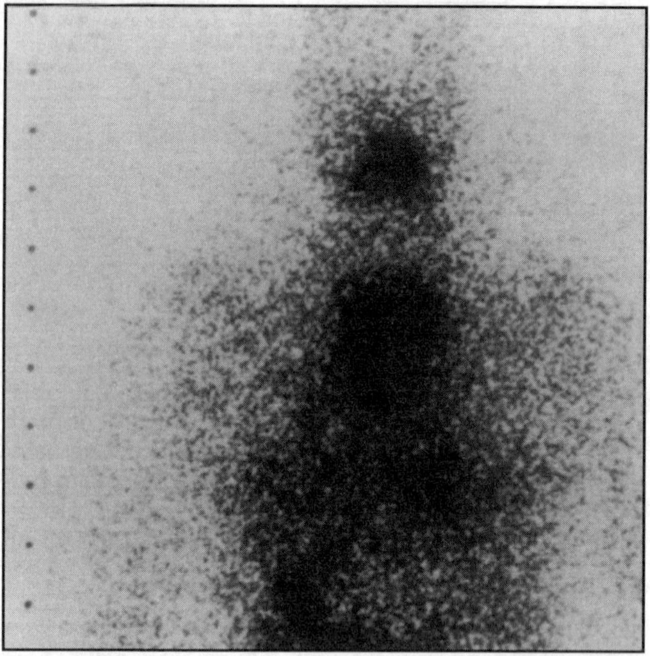

Figure 9-4: Metastatic thyroid carcinoma. Increased mediastinal and diffuse radioactivity in the lung fields bilaterally establish the presence of distant metastases in a patient with papillary/follicular carcinoma of the thyroid. Note the physiologic activity seen in the oral area above the neck, and in the stomach, below and to the left. (Used with permission, from: Sason JC: Selection of the optimal scanning agent for thyroid cancer. In: *Thyroid* 1997, pp 295-302).

The classical technique of whole body scanning after discontinuation of thyroxine often leads to severe symptomatology of hypothyroidism, including severe depression and even suicidal ideation. It is important for clinicians to understand that ^{131}I doses in excess of 3mCi (>111 MBq) may be associated with a *stunning* effect of the isotope on later applications of it for therapy. This may be caused by radiation imparted by the previous diagnostic ^{131}I that altered permeability of thyrocyte membranes. Because lower doses of ^{131}I make identification of small tumor foci less likely, however, a suitable intermediate schedule of no less than 2 mCi of ^{131}I (74 MBq) for diagnosis should permit adequate tissue sensitivity subsequently for treatment with ^{131}I (Figure 9-3).

Imaging of poorly differentiated papillary or follicular malignancies that do not concentrate ^{131}I is a challenging problem (Figure 9-4). Thallium 201 is a successful alternative agent for imaging thyroid and follicular carcinomas. The concentration of ^{201}Tl is related to blood flow to the tissue and concentration by thyroid tumor cells. ^{201}Tl concentrates in more than 50% of differentiated thyroid cancers, including Hürthle cell types.[3]

Other Imaging Radionuclides

Three other radioisotopic agents that may be concentrated in tumor tissues include ^{99}Tc-sestamibi, ^{99}Tc-tetrofosmin, and ^{111}Indium (^{111}In) octreotide, which is concentrated in most well-differentiated tumors, but also in tissues not imaged successfully with ^{131}I.

In the search for new radiopharmaceuticals for thyroid mass imaging, clinicians must consider the following paradox: if thyroid cancer is not visualized by ^{131}I imaging and the only treatment available is ^{131}I, what pharmacotherapies would be used in non-^{131}I imaged carcinomas?

Medullary Thyroid Carcinoma (MTC)

Medullary carcinomas, which originate in TCT cells and not in thyroid cells, are best localized with ^{111}In octreotide, but their identification does not lead to useful therapy. Re-operation for removal of MTC in cervical nodes has yielded conflicting results, and previous radionucleotide scans have not been used to enhance the outcomes of surgical procedures.

A recent novel therapy of MTC has been the application of ^{131}I-anti-carcinoembryonic antigen (CEA) antibodies, which require absorbed doses of radiation to be greater than the 5,000 cGy delivered by external beam irradiation, a goal that is difficult to obtain by ^{131}I antibody administration.[4] Moreover, because effective treatments of MTC are not yet available, the application of diagnostic imaging to localize metastatic MTC serves no purpose and is therefore not indicated.

Thyroid Ultrasonography

Ultrasound examination of the thyroid gland is very useful and inexpensive, noninvasive, causes no attendant tissue injuries, and does not require any isotopes or contrast materials to obtain a suitable image. Moreover, because the thyroid gland is near the skin surface, it can be seen almost completely except when tissue extends below the sternum. Sound waves are reflected differentially when acoustic impedance of tissues is different, such as the differences between solid masses and cystic masses. Solids are echoic, whereas cystic masses are characteristically anechoic.

Thyroid ultrasonography is used primarily to evaluate thyroid nodules to clarify whether they are cystic or solid, or complex with multiple septi. Also, high resolution of nodules as small as 1.5 cm can be achieved. However, ultrasound cannot determine if a nodule is benign or malignant. There are no unique ultrasonogram characteristics of thyroid carcinomas. Sonography of the thyroid gland is also helpful for guided needle biopsies of nonpalpable nodules. Finally, thyroid volume can be quantified accurately with this technology.

To perform ultrasonography, the patient is placed in a supine position, with the neck hyperextended. The ultrasound transducer is then pressed on the skin overlying the thyroid gland. A gel interface is required because sound waves do not pass readily through air alone. Typically, sagittal (longitudinal), axial (transverse), and oblique images are secured. Images can then be recorded on film or videotape.

In patients with known differentiated carcinoma of the thyroid, ultrasound is now the preferred method for detecting early recurrence, and 95% can be detected before masses become palpable. When a mass is palpated in the neck, ultrasound often allows the clinician to determine whether it extends from the thyroid gland or is separate from the thyroid gland, such as a lymph node. Finally, ultrasonography permits distinctions between solid (echoic) nodules and cystic structures, such as thyroglossal duct cysts.

References

1. Sostre S, Ashare AB, Quinones JD, et al: Thyroid scintigraphy: pinhole images versus rectilinear scans. *Radiology* 1978;129:759-762.

2. Greenspan FS, Strewler GJ, eds: The thyroid gland. In: *Basic and Clinical Endocrinology*. 5th ed. Stamford, Appleton & Lange, 1997.

3. Tonami N, Hisada K: 201ti scintigraphy in postoperative detection of thyroid cancer: a comparative study with ^{131}I. *Radiology* 1980;136:461-464.

4. Sisson JC: Selection of optimal scanning agent for thyroid cancer. *Thyroid* 1997;7:295-302.

Chapter 10

Illustrative Case Studies and Self-Assessment

Case 1

A 33-year-old woman was admitted to the hospital because of nervousness, sweating, hyperdefecation, and a 10-lb weight loss of 3 months' duration. She had been in good health before the onset of the illness. The patient reported a good appetite, but was experiencing up to 11 bowel movements per day. She noted weakness on stair climbing and rising from chairs.

On examination, the patient was thin and hyperkinetic, appearing younger than her age and in no acute distress. Her pulse was 120/minute and regular, blood pressure 130/60 mm Hg, respirations 22, and temperature 27.5° C. Her skin was warm and smooth, and she sweated profusely. The patient had no onycholysis but there was evidence of decreased proximal muscle strength. Her eyelids were retracted bilaterally, but there was no exophthalmos. Extraocular movements, visual fields, and vision were normal. The thyroid gland was diffusely enlarged and firmer than normal. Her heart was slightly enlarged with sinus tachycardia; her liver was palpable 1 fingerbreadth below the costal margin. No pretibial edema was found in her lower extremities. She demonstrated brisk symmetrical reflexes, and a tremor of the tongue and outstretched upper extremities.

Pertinent laboratory findings included hemoglobin 10.0 g/dL, hematocrit 33, and WBC of 4600/mm^3 with 38% polymorphonuclear leukocytes, 60% lymphocytes, and 2% monocytes. Chest x-ray was normal and the EKG showed tachycardia with tall T waves. Her serum cholesterol was 103 mg/dL.

Thyroid function test for this patient revealed:

T_4 = 16 μg/dL (normal 4 to 12)
T_3 uptake = 46% (normal 25 to 35)
T_3 (RIA) = 360 ng/dL (normal 90 to 20)
FT Index = 7.36 (normal 1.25 to 4.2)
TSH = <0.005 U/mL (normal 0.4 to 5.0)

Differential Diagnosis and Clinical Strategy

This patient has clinical signs and symptoms of thyrotoxicosis that most likely represent Graves' disease. However, because the patient has neither exophthalmos nor a bruit heard over the thyroid gland, the clinician must consider other causes of thyrotoxicosis, including transient thyrotoxicosis associated with chronic thyroiditis. To differentiate Graves' disease from chronic thyroiditis, a 24-hour radioactive ^{131}I uptake is indicated. In Graves' disease, the uptake would be markedly elevated, but would be extremely low or absent in chronic lymphocytic thyroiditis. In this patient, an extremely low thyroid uptake of 1% at 24 hours was obtained, indicating that management should be symptomatic with β-blockers. The administration of methimazole (Tapazole®) or propylthiouracil would be inappropriate and ineffectual. This syndrome should spontaneously resolve in a few months.

However, if the patient had demonstrated an elevated radioactive iodine uptake with an extremely low TSH—ruling out TSH-secreting tumor— a diagnosis of Graves' disease can be confirmed, particularly if antibodies to thyroglobulin and TPO are positive. Management in this instance would include β-blockers with antithyroid medication, either Tapazole® or propylthiouracil.

Case 2

A 59-year-old white female was hospitalized because of weakness, fatigue, poor memory, and cold intolerance of several years' duration. Two years before admission, the patient noted swelling of her ankles, shortness of breath, and anterior chest pain. She saw her family physician, who noted anemia (hematocrit 31), and prescribed a drug for angina, pentaerythritol (Peritrate®) and a diuretic (hydrochlorothiazide). The patient took these medications without apparent benefit for her malaise and weakness.

On physical examination, the patient had a low, hoarse voice, slowness of thought and movement, and a dull lethargy. In fact, she actually fell asleep twice during the medical history. Blood pressure was 140/70 mm Hg, pulse was 50/minute and regular, respirations were 16, and her temperature was 36.5° C. The patient's skin was thick, puffy, dry, and scaly. Scalp hair and eyebrow hair (lateral third) were reduced. The patient had impaired hearing. Her thyroid gland was diffusely enlarged 2x, and firm. There were no bruits heard over the thyroid. Lung examination was normal. Her heart was enlarged and heart sounds had diminished intensity. The skin on the extremities was thick, indurated, and dry (myxedema), with nonpitting edema to the knees. The heel pad callouses appeared orange. This coloration reflects impaired carotene to vitamin A conversion, which is thyroid and hormone dependent. The patient's cranial nerve functions were normal except for decrease in hearing. Deep tendon reflexes were symmetrically delayed in both contraction and relaxation phases. Her intellectual function was normal.

Laboratory work included hematocrit of 26% and hemoglobin of 8.5 g/dL. Urinalysis was normal. Chest x-ray revealed an enlarged heart. An echocardiogram revealed sinus rhythm, with pericardial effusion. The EKG showed low voltage with diffuse ST and T wave changes. The serum T_4 was 2 g/dL (normal = 4.5 to 12), and the serum TSH was 84 U/mL.

Differential Diagnosis and Clinical Strategy

This patient had hypothyroidism, associated with a goiter and accelerated atherogenesis, as reflected by angina pectoris and heart failure. Additional laboratory studies revealed a serum thyroxine concentration of 1.4 g/dL, below normal, with an elevated TSH of 84 U/mL. In the presence of thyroid tissue, the clinician can exclude hypothyroidism caused by previous radioiodine therapy for Graves' disease or for thyroid surgery. Congential causes, such as blockade of iodide organification in the thyroid gland, were not reasonable diagnoses in this patient because of her normal adult height and the absence of impaired intellectual development during childhood. The most common cause of painless hypothyroidism associated with goiter in the United States is chronic lymphocytic thyroiditis (Hashimoto's disease). This diagnosis can be confirmed by demonstrating antibodies to thyroglobulin and to TPO.

Appropriate therapy in this case was administration of graduated oral thyroxin beginning at 0.025 mg/day, with the dosage gradually doubling every 4 weeks to 0.1 mg/day. Further elevations should then be made until a final T_4 dosage is reached between 0.112 and 0.15 mg/day. Fluids were administered cautiously. The patient was greatly improved at discharge.

If primary hypothyroidism occurs in a young patient without evidence of coronary disease, a near complete replacement therapy with thyroxine can be begun immediately, starting at 0.1 mg/day.

Clinical Thyroidology: Self-Assessment Thyroid Case Studies

Use the following material to test your clinical understanding of thyroid disorders. The answers are at the end of each quiz section.

In the first test, match the thyroid laboratory profile (a through e) with the patient profile.

	Total T_4 (μg/dL)	Free T_4 (μg/dL)	Total T_3 (ng/mL)	TSH (μU/mL)	24-hour ^{131}I update (%)
(a)	17.1	3.8	288	<0.01	<1
(b)	9.1	1.6	126	1.6	17
(c)	4.3	0.46	102	0.22	<1
(d)	4.1	0.6	101	27.7	6
(e)	22.2	4.1	650	<0.01	65

1. A 19-year-old woman 5 weeks postpartum has a depressed mood, marked fatigue, and lethargy.
2. A 65-year-old woman presents with a large thyroid incidentaloma found on annual examination, 3 x 4 cm, firm, nontender. She has no complaints. A thyroid scan shows a nonfunctioning nodule, highly echogenic on ultrasound. A FNA showed cells suspicious for malignancy.
3. A 22-year-old female presented with 3 weeks of heat intolerance and intense neck tenderness over the thyroid region. She has recently had an URI. PE revealed sinus tachycardia and a diffusely enlarged, exquisitely tender thyroid gland.
4. A 47-year-old woman with a new diagnosis of atrial fibrillation reported anxiousness and tremulousness. PE revealed tachycardia, ophthalmopathy, and a diffusely enlarged, nontender thyroid gland.

5. A 51-year-old man with headache, lethargy, hoarseness, and peripheral vision loss.

Answers: (1) d, (2) b, (3) a, (4) e (5) c

In the next test, determine the correct diagnosis based on the patient profile.

1. A 45-year-old was admitted for acute pneumonitis and fever and required mechanical ventilation for 5 days. On a battery of tests, T_4 level was found to be below normal at 3.4 (normal = 4.5 to 12). Follow-up tests showed a TT_3 of 40 ng/dL (normal = 100 to 200). The TSH was 0.7 U/mL. What is your diagnosis and what laboratory test may clinch it?
2. A 37-year-old obese woman had palpitations, anxiety, and insomnia. Examination disclosed a pulse of 120. Neck examination revealed no palpable thyroid. She has failed multiple previous diet attempts, including dexfenfluramine. What is your differential diagnosis and what laboratory test may help in verifying your diagnosis?
3. A 38-year-old woman presented for follow-up. She is taking L-T_4 (0.125 mg/day PO) for Hashimoto's thyroiditis. The free T_4 is normal, but, the TSH is 12.8 U/mL. What is your recommendation at this point?
4. A 38-year-old male with nephrotic syndrome had complaints of malaise. A total T_4 test was abnormally low at 3.6 g/dL. However, serum TSH test was normal. You suspect that this abnormality may be caused by his nephrotic syndrome. What would the T_3 resin uptake or free T_4 show?

Answers:

(1) Euthyroid sick syndrome. Measurement of reverse T_3 (rT_3) will confirm elevation of rT_3.

(2) Thyrotoxicosis factitia. The key finding is the serum Tg, which is low. It is elevated in thyroid gland causes of thyrotoxicosis.

(3) This probably represents noncompliance, a very common syndrome. If the patient took T_4 correctly only in the last few days, T_4 would be normalized, but TSH would still be elevated.

(4) An elevated T_3 resin uptake is due to low serum binding of thyroid hormones. TBG, TBPA, and albumin are lost in the urine, which lowers the total T_4. Free T_4 would be normal, and the patient should be euthyroid clinically.

Index

D

E

I

J

K

L

M

N

O

P

R

U

V

W

Notes